2OX3
ELIMINATE YOUR BELLY FAT
IN AN HOUR A WEEK

Dr Steve Boutcher is an associate professor at the School of Medical Sciences at the University of New South Wales. With a special interest in healthy weight loss, he has spent 10 years researching the best way to get maximum benefit from nutrition and exercise, and this ground-breaking book is the result.

20 X 3

ELIMINATE YOUR BELLY FAT IN AN HOUR A WEEK

DR STEVE BOUTCHER

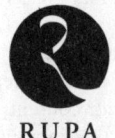

RUPA

Published by
Rupa Publications India Pvt. Ltd 2014
7/16, Ansari Road, Daryaganj
New Delhi 110002

Sales centres:
Allahabad Bengaluru Chennai
Hyderabad Jaipur Kathmandu
Kolkata Mumbai

Copyright © Dr Steve Boutcher 2013

First published in Australia by Nero,
an imprint of Schwartz Media Pty Ltd in 2013

This edition published by arrangement with the original publisher.

While every effort has been made to verify the authenticity of the
information contained in this book, it is not intended as a substitute for
medical consultation with a physician. The publisher and the author are in
no way liable for the use of the information contained in this book.

All rights reserved.
No part of this publication may be reproduced, transmitted, or
stored in a retrieval system, in any form or by any means, electronic,
mechanical, photocopying, recording or otherwise, without the prior
permission of the publisher.

ISBN: 978-81-291-3134-8

First impression 2014

10 9 8 7 6 5 4 3 2 1

The moral right of the author has been asserted.

This edition is for sale in the Indian Subcontinent only.

Printed at Replika Press Pvt. Ltd., India

This book is sold subject to the condition that it shall not, by way
of trade or otherwise, be lent, resold, hired out, or otherwise circulated,
without the publisher's prior consent, in any form of binding or
cover other than that in which it is published.

Contents

Introduction	1
1. Understanding belly fat	5
2. The effect of exercise on belly fat and health	34
3. The interval sprinting belly fat loss program	75
4. Dieting, nutrients and belly fat	113
5. Reducing daily stress and enhancing sleep quality	162
6. A 6-week belly fat loss program	189
Appendices	200
Acknowledgements	215
Resources	216
Endnotes	220
Index	231

Introduction

The human body is programmed to store fat for a number of reasons but the places it stores fat have different effects on our health. Fat under the skin on our legs and arms is considered a healthy fat and helps to prevent diseases such as type 2 diabetes. In contrast, visceral or belly fat clusters around our internal organs and has been found to contribute to the development of diabetes and cardiovascular and inflammatory diseases. This is because the fat in the belly is released to the liver, which affects the way your body reacts to insulin and eventually leads to decreased insulin sensitivity, potentially causing type 2 diabetes and leading to other serious diseases.

Factors such as age, gender, genes and lifestyle all influence the amount of fat that is deposited around the organs in your belly; for example, postmenopausal women typically have greater belly fat stores than younger women. Similarly, older men tend to have more belly fat than young men. It has also been discovered that people of Asian descent who experience increases in belly fat have a greater incidence of cardiovascular problems than non-Asians. People who are under stress and those who sleep poorly also tend to have more belly fat. And, of course, those individuals who consume a lot of junk food and excessive alcohol and do little exercise typically possess greater belly fat stores.

Our research has found that an interval sprinting program, combined with a healthy Mediterranean eating plan, is the most effective way to reduce dangerous belly fat. The program we have developed has been scientifically shown to improve overall health in much less time than conventional exercise programs like jogging and weight training. Our interval sprinting program recommends exercising for 20 minutes a session, 3 times per week – a total of about 1 hour of exercise a week. By exercising for only 1 hour a week, you can reduce your belly and body fat, as well as increase the muscle mass in your legs and abdomen, which is important for prevention of type 2 diabetes. Interval sprinting has also been proven to significantly reduce insulin resistance – the key for long-term health – and improve cardiovascular health within just 6 weeks.

Combining the interval sprinting program with a healthy Mediterranean eating plan and consumption of foods proven to have a beneficial effect on health, like green tea, can extend the health benefits of interval sprinting. Of course, if you begin an interval sprinting program but continue to eat in an unhealthy manner, then the positive effects of the exercise will be prevented or reduced.

Eating healthy foods and participating in a well-structured interval sprinting program can significantly reduce your belly fat and improve your health. This book will show you how.

How to use this book

This book contains:

- The interval sprinting program to help you lose belly fat, increase aerobic fitness and muscle mass, and reduce insulin resistance;

- Information about healthy eating and what nutrients to ingest before and after sprinting exercise for the best results; and

- A guide to reducing the effect of daily stressors and enhancing sleep quality to prevent an increase in belly fat.

By following the advice and methods in this book, you can significantly reduce your belly fat and improve your health. Chapter 1 explains why belly fat is so dangerous to ongoing good health, how it accumulates and how to determine whether you are carrying a dangerous amount of belly fat. Chapter 2 explains how interval sprinting can help reduce belly fat and increase overall health, and the types of exercises suited to interval sprinting and the program itself are covered in Chapter 3. Chapters 4 and 5 show you how to apply the exercise, healthy eating and stress-management program to your life. Finally, Chapter 6 offers a sample plan for you to follow to lose belly fat and improve your health.

Chapter 1
Understanding belly fat

Australians are getting fatter and more obese – we now rank in the top 5 fattest nations on earth and have the second highest rate of childhood obesity.[1] During the last 100 years, overweight and obesity rates of Australian children have escalated: in the early 1900s, the overweight and obesity rate in Australian children was around 6% but today it is about 30%, and this rise is predicted to continue. This pattern is common in the majority of developed countries, such as the USA and Europe. In the USA, over a third of adults (36%) are currently obese, while in the United Kingdom the number of obese adults increased from 16% to 24% in women and from 13% to 22% in men between 1993 and 2009. There is also potential for a dramatic increase in obesity rates in developing areas such as India, the Middle East and Asia, as overweight and obesity rates in those regions have escalated during the last twenty years.[2]

An increase in dangerous belly fat is also happening, as demonstrated by the increase in average waist circumferences around the world. Having a waist circumference less than 80cm for women and 94cm for men is recommended for health reasons, but in the USA the average waist circumference went from 89cm in 1962 to 99cm in 2000 in men, and from 77cm to 94cm in women.[3] Another study in the USA monitored over 100,000 middle-aged men and women over 9 years. Results showed that, compared to people with a normal waist size, people with large waists – greater than 120cm for men and 110cm for women – had about twice the early death rate.[4] In the UK, a 2011 study found that the average waist circumference of young girls, 71cm, was 13cm bigger than girls of the same age measured 30 years previously.[5]

As world levels of belly fat increase, so does the incidence of type 2 diabetes and cardiovascular disease, so it's important we understand why we are putting on belly fat and how we can stop this trend.

What is fat?

We have a layer of fat under the skin called subcutaneous fat. This fat makes up about 80–90% of our total body fat and is typically located on the back of the arms, below the shoulder blades, around the belly and on the upper legs and hips. The remaining 10–20% of our body fat is termed belly fat, also known as visceral fat, and is located beneath the stomach muscles and around internal organs such as the liver, spleen, intestines and kidneys. In some people, belly fat can also accumulate in organs such as the liver. Interestingly, people who have more fat on their upper thighs have less incidence of type 2 diabetes and cardiovascular disease.[6]

Subcutaneous fat serves a number of purposes, such as keeping us warm and acting as a storage site for hormones and energy. Also called adipose tissue, it used to be thought of mainly as a ready source of energy in times of famine, but fat is now viewed as an endocrine organ that stores and excretes a number of hormones and chemicals that can have both positive and negative effects on health. Fat mass secretes over 30 chemical messengers; some messengers, such as the hormone leptin, tell the brain that we have had enough to eat, whereas other chemicals, such as tumour necrosis factor, a cytokine, induce inflammation to help to combat pathogens.

Too much inflammation, however, results in cardiovascular disease and insulin resistance. High levels of these inflammatory chemicals can result in a reduction in cellular insulin sensitivity and eventually insulin resistance, which occurs when the muscle and liver cells become unresponsive to insulin in the blood. Insulin comes from the pancreas and carries the sugar in the blood to the cells of the body, and high levels of insulin and glucose in the blood increase the risk of type

2 diabetes. People with type 2 diabetes typically have excessive belly fat, high blood pressure and elevated blood triglyceride levels. Fat cells also secrete a chemical called adiponectin, which has anti-diabetic properties.

We all possess billions of fat cells but it has been shown that an absolute fat cell number is established during the teenage years, and this remains constant during adulthood. One study that assessed genomic DNA was able to retrospectively measure fat cell number in humans.[7] Both obese and lean children established their peak fat cell number during adolescence, with little change occurring during adulthood. Importantly, those who became obese during adolescence possessed billions more fat cells than their leaner counterparts. As the fat cell lasts about 8 to 10 years, any extra fat cells children develop increase their fat storage capacity, which leads to obesity development, and overweight teenagers will therefore have those billions of extra fat cells for the rest of their lives.

Visceral or belly fat is different from subcutaneous fat and is much more dangerous, as it contributes to type 2 diabetes, cardiovascular and inflammatory disease.[8] As can be seen in Figure 1, belly fat lies underneath the tummy muscles. As belly fat is firmer than subcutaneous fat, it pushes the abdominal muscles outward. These fat cells reside deep in the abdomen and consequently do not release their fatty acids into the circulation but deliver them straight to the liver. Too many fatty acids released to the liver make the liver produce other forms of fat, called triglyceride and cholesterol, which are then secreted into the circulation. High levels of triglycerides and cholesterol in our blood are bad for health.

Belly fat cells also have a greater blood supply than subcutaneous fat cells, and thus can release fatty acids and hormones far more quickly. The good news is that, compared to subcutaneous fat cells, belly fat cells are far more responsive to circulating catecholamines. These are the major hormones for fat release and fat burning and can be significantly elevated by interval sprinting exercise, as discussed in Chapter 3. This means belly fat is easier to lose than subcutaneous fat.

How belly fat accumulates

Belly fat accumulation is influenced by a number of factors, such as possessing high levels of fat-storing hormones and low levels of fat-burning hormones, being sedentary and having certain genes. Eating too much processed food is also related to belly fat accumulation and is covered in more detail in Chapter 4. Other factors affecting belly fat accumulation include age, ethnicity and lifestyle.

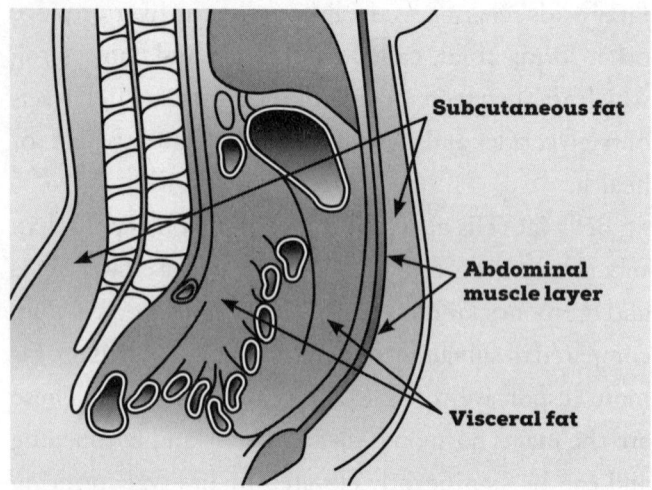

Figure 1. Abdominal stores of subcutaneous and belly fat (visceral fat).

Fat-storing hormones

Cortisol, a hormone that is secreted into the blood by the adrenal glands, is typically elevated when people experience stress. When blood cortisol levels increase, the amount of sugar in the blood also increases, which results in a corresponding rise in insulin. Having elevated levels of cortisol and insulin in the blood encourages fat storage and impedes fat burning. This means high levels of stress increase the levels of cortisol and insulin in your blood, leading to reduced fat release and increased belly fat stores. Cortisol may also contribute to leptin resistance, which means people eat more, as leptin is a satiety hormone that fat cells release to tell the brain we have had enough to eat.

Fat-burning hormones

In humans, catecholamines are the major hormones that mobilise fat from fat cells and induce fat burning in muscles and the liver. The catecholamines are epinephrine (or adrenalin) and norepinpehrine (or noradrenalin) and are secreted into the blood by the adrenal glands. Norepinephrine is also released at nerve endings. Blood catecholamine levels gradually increase through the night and typically peak around 11am. Catecholamine-induced fat mobilisation occurs much more in belly fat compared to subcutaneous fat.

Unfortunately, this catecholamine-induced release of fat is suppressed in obese individuals. This suppression occurs at a young age as it is present in obese teenagers and in obese children, whose mobilisation of triglyceride stores by epinephrine was decreased by 30% during rest. This inability to mobilise lipids increases the amount of fat depots in our bodies and can lead to abdominal obesity. Its cause is undetermined but appears to be influenced by defective fat cell receptors.

Another fat-burning hormone is growth hormone, which is produced by the pituitary gland. Insulin slows down growth hormone release, so people with high levels of insulin in their blood typically have lower levels of growth hormone. Having problems with the thyroid gland can also result in increased belly fat accumulation. The thyroid is an endocrine gland located at the base of the neck and releases a hormone called T3 (thyroid hormone), which elevates metabolic rate and, together with catecholamines and growth hormone, increases fat release from cells. Hypothyroidism occurs when the thyroid gland produces too little T3 or the thyroid receptors in cells become insensitive. Low thyroid levels can contribute to elevated fat deposition and can cause an increase in belly fat stores and are often accompanied by elevated low-grade inflammation, as hypothyroid individuals have been shown to possess increased levels of C-reactive protein, an inflammatory chemical, in their blood.

Genetic influences

Over the last 3 decades, researchers have discovered genetic markers that contribute to increased body weight and waist circumference, however no single gene has been found to cause obesity. Specific genes related to obesity have been identified; among them are a number of single gene mutations that contribute to the development of obesity in teenagers and young adults. This means we now know that genes affect belly fat development when influenced by factors such as physical inactivity, nutrient intake and metabolic status.

Lifestyle factors that influence belly fat accumulation

There are many lifestyle factors that impact on belly fat, but perhaps the most important (after eating and exercise) are age, drinking alcohol, ethnicity, smoking, stress and sleep. Exposure to daily stressors and reduced quality of sleep have both been associated with belly fat accumulation. Chapter 5 covers how poor sleep and uncontrolled daily stress can lead to belly fat development, together with a description of stress-management and sleep-enhancing techniques.

Physical inactivity
People who do not do recreational exercise and have little physical activity in their jobs are prone to belly fat accumulation, especially if they consume a lot of processed food. This belly fat accumulation risks developing cardiovascular disease, as well as type 2 diabetes. Exercising burns up energy and gradually makes the body metabolise more fat than carbohydrate. It is also likely that fat burning continues during the period after exercise. See Chapter 2 for a discussion of how different forms of exercise have differing effects on body fat and muscle mass.

Genes play a role in aerobic fitness levels, and estimates of their contribution to such fitness vary between 10% and 40%: if you have parents who were good at

Answer the questions with regard to your typical weekly physical activity patterns. Fill in a score between 1 and 4 for each question and then sum your total.

1 = Not at all **2 = Sometimes**
3 = Fairly regularly **4 = All the time**

1. I exercise (walk, run, cycle, swim) at least 3 times per week
2. My exercise sessions last for at least 30 minutes
3. When I exercise I breathe heavily and sweat
4. My daily job involves a lot of physical activity
5. I do a lot of housework and gardening
6. During my recreation time I do a lot of physical activity

TOTAL

Interpreting your score:

6-9 points: low levels of physical activity
10-12 points: moderately low levels of physical activity
13-18 points: moderately high levels of physical activity
19-24 points: high levels of physical activity

activities such as cross-country running, it is likely that you will carry genes that will make you good at performing aerobic running exercise. However, all kinds of fitness are mainly influenced by exercising, and to keep fit you need to perform physical activity.

Exercise physiologists assess people's aerobic fitness by exercising them to exhaustion on a bike or treadmill and measuring their maximum oxygen uptake, which reflects aerobic fitness. Assessing maximum oxygen uptake, however, requires expertise and expensive equipment. An easier way of assessing aerobic fitness is to see how far you can walk or run on level ground in 12 minutes. This test is called the Cooper 12-minute walk/run fitness test and is described in Appendix A, on page 200.[9]

On page 14 is a questionnaire assessment that does not involve exercising. If you score 9 points or less on the questionnaire, or walk or run less than 1 kilometre on the walk/run fitness test, it is likely that you are really unfit and need to begin a fitness program.

Age

Older people tend to have more belly fat than young people. The main reason for the increase in belly fat in older people seems to be a decrease in the body's metabolism: after the age of 30, most people's metabolism will decrease about 1% every 2 years. Why metabolism slows down as we age is unclear, but it probably involves a decrease in muscle mass and a change in hormone levels. While the amount of subcutaneous fat generally declines with ageing, so does muscle mass, and since skeletal muscles, together with the liver, are the major fat burning engines of the body, older people burn lower levels of fat overall.

The decrease in muscle mass with ageing, however, is not inevitable, as people who perform regular weight training typically retain most of their muscle mass and ability to lift weights. Thus, decreased muscle mass with ageing for most people occurs because they are not challenging their skeletal muscles regularly. The good news is that interval sprinting exercise can significantly increase muscle mass.

As we age, blood hormone levels can decrease because of reduced secretion by the body's endocrine glands. The receptors on the body's cells can become insensitive too and don't respond to hormones effecttively. For women, the largest hormonal change concerns decreased oestrogen when menopause occurs, whereas for men, the largest hormonal change typically involves reduced testosterone.

Alcohol

Alcohol contains 7 calories per gram which is more than the 5 calories contained in a gram of carbohydrate and protein and just under the 9 calories per gram contained in fat. Thus, consuming 2–3 average-sized alcoholic drinks a day adds up to over 500 calories. In a week, over 3500 extra calories would be consumed. Since 1 calorie equals 9 grams of fat, that means having 3 drinks every day of the week adds almost 400g of fat to your diet. According to studies in this area, the majority of these calories appear to be deposited as belly fat. It has also been shown that consuming alcohol makes people hungry.

However, a small amount of daily beer or wine, containing 14 grams of ethanol for women and about 28 grams for men, is beneficial for health. An average drink – a regular-sized glass of beer or wine – contains about 14 grams of ethanol. Studies have shown that women who drink about 1 drink a day and men who consume 2 drinks a day have a lower incidence of diabetes, stroke and heart disease.[9]

Ethnicity

Surprising differences emerge when belly fat accumulation is compared between different ethnicities. A study conducted by Louisiana State University researchers found similar results to a number of other studies that have shown that African-American women possessed less belly fat compared to Caucasian women.[10] A research study of African-American and Caucasian men involving universities from Canada and the USA showed similar results.[11] An article published in the *International Journal of Obesity* also indicated that Japanese-American men had greater amounts of belly fat than Caucasian men.[12]

However, the strongest relationship between negative health and accumulation of belly fat seems to occur in people of South Asian descent. Research conducted at the State University of New York found high amounts of belly fat in Indian migrants, although they were not obese.[13] A study by Canadian researchers in 2011 found that people of South Asian descent accumulated dangerous belly fat on and in their internal organs when they put on total body fat. Adding belly fat to and inside organs like the liver and kidneys is more likely to lead to coronary artery disease and type 2 diabetes. In contrast, people of Caucasian descent added fat to their waistline rather than deep inside their bellies.[14] These researchers also found that people who originated from India, even though they possessed a similar BMI to Caucasians, had significantly more belly fat. They also had more cardiovascular disease risk factors, such as metabolic syndrome and high cholesterol levels. The researchers suggested that, compared to people of Caucasian descent, those with South Asian heritage had less room underneath their skin to store fat (subcutaneous fat), therefore their excess fat was stored in fat compartments deep in the belly.

Overall, the increase in belly fat appears to be particularly troublesome in people of South Asian descent, as they seem to suffer more health problems, such as atherosclerosis and type 2 diabetes, when they develop belly fat. This is why the BMI cut-off for health problems by being overweight sometimes differs by ethnicities (see Table 1, page 24).

Why small increases in belly fat in people of Asian descent bring about greater cardiovascular problems than in non-Asians is unclear. Why people with South Asian heritage are getting fatter, however, is likely due to a change in lifestyle. People of Asian compared to European ethnicity have typically possessed far less body and belly obesity, an outcome of their plant-based diets and physically active lifestyle. However, developing countries such as India and China are now adopting Westernised lifestyles that involve consuming much more processed food and performing far less physical activity. The outcome is that countries that used to have very low levels of obesity and type 2 diabetes now have the fastest growth rates of these diseases. Given that developing countries are rapidly adopting Westernised lifestyles and that many Asians who emigrate eat Western foods and do not exercise, it is very important for individuals of Asian ethnicity to prevent an increase in belly fat by eating healthy foods and exercising regularly.

Smoking

Typically, smokers weigh less than non-smokers, as smoking may reduce appetite and also elevate metabolic rate, which induces fat burning. There is evidence, however, to show that cigarette smoking increases belly fat accumulation: a large, population-based study in the UK found that men and women who smoked possessed increased belly fat.[15] How smoking increases belly fat is unclear, but shortly after a smoker finishes a cigarette, blood cortisol levels can increase for up to 30 minutes. We know that cortisol can increase belly fat accumulation due to its effect on blood sugar and insulin levels. Smokers also exercise far less than non-smokers, which is also likely to contribute to increased belly fat accumulation.

The impact of belly fat on health

As mentioned, belly fat emits a number of chemicals that can negatively affect health. Belly fat cells secrete chemicals called cytokines, which make the liver inflamed. They also bombard the liver with free fatty acids, which are converted to triglyceride and cholesterol and end up in the bloodstream. This cycle can cause type 2 diabetes and lead to atherosclerosis and cardiovascular disease.

Increased belly fat has been associated with a number of medical conditions, including:

- cardiovascular disease
- type 2 diabetes
- hypertension

- elevated blood cholesterol
- increased blood sugar
- dementia
- asthma
- colorectal cancer
- breast cancer
- bowel cancer
- pancreatic cancer
- endometriosis
- gallbladder problems
- sleep apnoea

For example, in Chinese adults, a bigger waist circumference – an indicator of belly fat – predicted development of hypertension, regardless of whether a person was normal weight or overweight.[16] Another study found that older people with more belly fat had worse memories and were less verbally fluent.[17] Interestingly, researchers from Spain tracked 3235 adult men and women for 2 years and found that waist circumference predicted disability. People with the largest waist circumference had 2.2 times more risk of mobility disability and 4.8 times more agility disability compared to adults with lower waist circumference.[18] And a study in Europe involving nearly half a million women found that excessive belly fat, estimated by waist-to-hip ratio, was related to elevated colorectal cancer risk.[19]

Possessing elevated levels of body and belly fat increases general cancer risk, and people with large waistlines are at higher risk for bowel, breast and pancreatic cancer development and, in postmenopausal women, for cancer of the womb lining. Studies have also shown that in both young and older Japanese-American men, belly fat obesity predicted heart attack and hypertension development. Belly fat accumulation has also been associated with gallstones and Alzheimer's disease.

How to measure your body and belly fat

Measuring body fat accurately is difficult. To measure body fat, medical professionals and researchers use methods that include magnetic resonance imaging (MRI), dual energy X-ray absorptiometry (DEXA), computed tomography, underwater weighing, skinfolds, Bod Pod (a volume-measuring technique) and bioelectrical impedance (opposition to the flow of an electrical current through the body). Unfortunately, most of these methods are expensive, and DEXA and computed tomography involve ionising radiation. These assessments all have their strengths and weaknesses but all incur a cost. Low-cost indirect measures, such as body mass index (BMI), provide an approximate estimate of body fat.

BMI

BMI is calculated by dividing a person's body weight in kilograms by their height in metres squared. BMI has been used to identify individuals whose weight increases their risk for heart disease and diabetes. People with BMIs of 25.0 to 29.9kg per square metre (kg/m^2) are considered overweight, and those with BMIs of 30kg/m^2 are considered obese. However, BMI can be misleading because it does not consider muscle mass, so very muscular or tall individuals can have a BMI of over 30kg/m^2 but actually can be very lean. To calculate your BMI, go to www.health.gov.au/internet/healthyactive/publishing.nsf/Content/your-bmi, or use the formula below.

How to calculate your BMI
Divide your weight in kilograms by your height squared in metres. A male weighing 85 kilograms with a height of 1.8 metres, for example, would first multiply 1.8 metres by 1.8 metres to get 3.24 metres, then divide 85 kilograms by 3.24 metres to arrive at a BMI of 26 (that is, 26kg/m^2).

As can be seen in Table 1, a BMI of greater than 25 is considered overweight, whereas a BMI of 30 and over

Classification	Cut off points for non-Asians
Underweight	<18.5
Severe thinness	<16.0
Moderate thinness	16.0–16.9
Mild thinness	17.0–18.5
Normal range	18.5–24.9
Overweight	>25.0
Pre-obese	25.0–29.9
Obese	<30.0
Obese class I	30.0–34.9
Obese class II	35.0–39.9
Obese class III	>40.0

Table 1. Criteria for body mass index (BMI) in adults (BMI = weight ÷ height squared).

Adapted from The International Classification of Adult Underweight, Overweight and Obesity according to BMI.[20]

is obese. BMI values are independent of age for adults, and although BMI is the same for both genders, it varies according to ethnicity. The World Health Organisation convened the Expert Consultation on BMI in Asian populations in 2002 and concluded that the number of Asians with a high risk of type 2 diabetes and cardiovascular disease was substantially more at BMIs lower than the existing WHO cut-off point for overweight,

25kg/m². The BMI cut-off point for increased moderate health risk ranged from 22 to 25 in different Asian populations, and ranged from 26 to 31 for high health risk. In Japan and China a BMI of greater than 23 is now considered overweight and an increased health risk.

Bioelectrical impedance devices

Bioelectrical impedance analysis devices are relatively cheap but tend to underestimate body fat. Although their results are affected by the amount of water found in bodily tissues, if used regularly under standardised conditions – once a week, fasting in the morning – they will give a reasonable estimate of body fat change. Optimal body fat levels have been suggested to be around 10–20% in men and 20–25% in women.

A new bioelectrical impedance device for measuring belly or visceral fat has recently been developed by Tanita and is called the Viscan AB 140. Comparisons between this device and estimates of central fat carried out by DEXA have shown that their values are very similar (they correlate about r=0.95). However, comparisons between gold-standard estimates of belly fat such as MRI and computed tomography do not appear to have been carried out.

Risk category	Gender	Waist circumference
Europid	Men Women	>94cm >80cm
South Asian	Men Women	>90cm >80cm
Chinese	Men Women	>90cm >80cm
Japanese	Men Women	>90cm >80cm

Table 2. International Diabetes Federation criteria for ethnic or country-specific values for waist circumference.

Adapted from Alberti, Zimmet and Shaw.[21]

Waist circumference

Waist circumference is an easy measure to obtain and is strongly related to belly fat assessed by clinical methods. Thus, having a large waist circumference usually means you have a significant amount of belly fat. Measure your waist circumference immediately above your navel with the tape being level with the top of your right hip bone. The tape measure should not be pulled too tight and you should take shallow breaths. Having someone else take the measure reduces error, and it is best if 2 measurements are taken and the average value recorded. Optimal waist circumferences for men and women of Asian and European descent are indicated in Table 2 on page 26, but if you are very large or tall these values may be inaccurate. Waist circumference greater than these values is associated with increased cardiovascular and metabolic health problems.

Abdominal width

Belly fat tends to remain in the same position in your abdomen whether you are standing up or lying down. In contrast, abdominal subcutaneous fat – the fat you can pinch around your tummy – will tend to move sideways and downwards when in a lying position. To test if you have a lot of belly fat, you can compare your abdominal width when you are standing up and lying down.

Stand against a wall, making sure to push your spine against it. Place something flat, such as a plastic ruler, across your abdomen, then use a tape measure or another ruler to measure your abdominal width from the wall to the plastic ruler. Record the distance. Now lie on a flat surface. Place the ruler on your abdomen and measure from floor to ruler with the tape measure. If the measurement does not change much and if you have a large waist circumference (as per the measurements in Table 2), then it is likely you possess a lot of belly fat. If the difference is large – a 2.5cm difference can be considered large – you probably have a significant amount of subcutaneous abdominal fat.

These simple methods will not assess exactly how much belly fat you possess but they will let you know if interval sprinting is reducing your belly fat over time. If you undertake the program described in Chapter 6, measuring abdominal width and waist circumference weekly are good ways of assessing your progress.

Waist skinfold measure

An estimate of total body fat can also be achieved by measuring the thickness of skinfolds in different parts of the body. This is done with a device called a skinfold calliper, which assesses the thickness of the skin together with a layer of subcutaneous fat. Taking skinfolds at different parts of the body can give you an estimate of the amount of subcutaneous fat on your body. Formulas have been developed to estimate the total percentage of body fat from calliper measurements, however the accuracy of these has been questioned. Like bioelectrical impedance, calliper measurements are best used to estimate subcutaneous fat change over time rather than one single estimate of total body fat.

Skinfold assessment does not estimate belly fat, however it can be used to monitor changes in the subcutaneous fat around your belly. A useful place to take a measurement is the waist skinfold, which is illustrated in Figure 2 on page 29. The waist, or suprailiac, skinfold is located just above the protrusion of the hip bone,

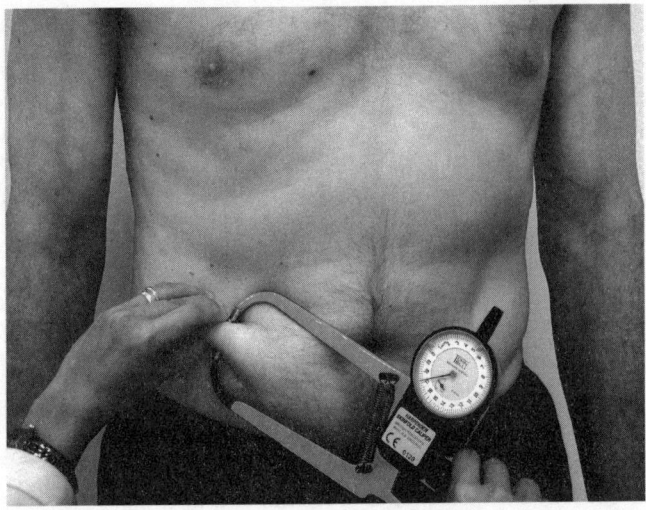

Figure 2. Assessment of waist subcutaneous fat by skinfold.

which is known as the iliac crest. It is more accurate if you get someone else to do the measurement for you. It is important that the skinfold is taken in the same position every time. Taking a picture of the site with a digital camera is recommended.

The fold is taken almost horizontally. For right-handed people, pinch and hold a fold of skin with its layer of subcutaneous fat with the left forefinger and thumb. Using the right hand, place the calliper jaws about 8mm from the left forefinger. Keep holding the skinfold with the left hand throughout. Release the calliper so all the force of its jaws is on the skinfold alone. The callipers will take a few moments to stabilise; the value should

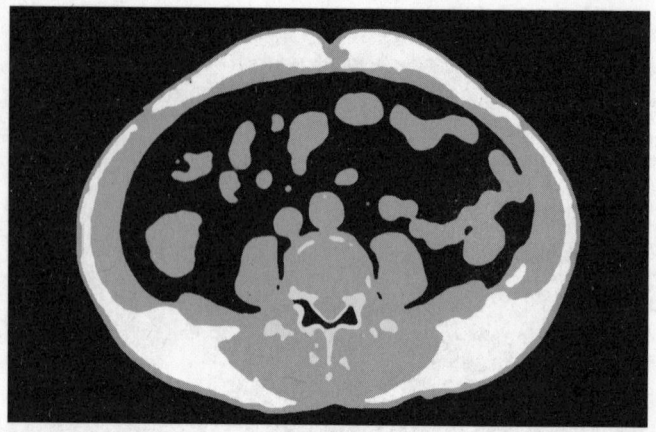

Figure 3. A computed tomography scan across the waist area. White is the subcutaneous abdominal fat, grey is mostly abdominal muscle and other tissue, and black is the belly, or visceral, fat.

only be recorded when they have stopped changing and before releasing any calliper pressure. Measure the waist site twice and record the readings on the Body Composition Recording Form (see Appendix E, page 208).

*

Now you have 3 abdominal and belly fat measures that can be used to monitor subcutaneous and belly fat change as you proceed with the interval sprinting program:

- waist circumference

- abdominal width

- waist skinfold

In Figure 3 (on page 30), the subcutaneous abdominal fat is shown in white, the abdominal muscle in grey, and the belly or visceral fat in black. If your waist circumference gets smaller, then either your subcutaneous abdominal fat (white) or belly fat (black) has been reduced. If your waist circumference gets smaller but the skinfold caliper measure does not change then it is likely that your belly fat has decreased.

How to measure leg circumference

Measuring skeletal muscle mass is best done through clinical techniques such as MRI and DEXA. For individual monitoring, however, the assessment of leg circumferences can provide an indirect guide to possible change in muscle mass after interval sprinting. Leg measurements are obtained in a similar fashion to waist circumference, and are taken at mid-thigh and at the widest point of the calf.

For the mid-thigh measurement, use a tape measure to assess the distance between your groin and the top of your kneecap, and then determine the mid-point of the measurement. You should mark the site with a non-permanent ink pen and take a digital picture to ensure you measure in the same place each time. Stand with your weight evenly distributed on both feet and wrap the tape measure around the mid-point of your thigh. The tape measure should not be pulled too tight.

Having someone else take the measurement reduces error, and it is best if 2 measures are recorded and the average value documented. Record the results on the Body Composition Recording Form (see Appendix E, page 208).

*

The key points to remember about the problems of having too much belly fat are:

- **Worldwide, belly fat accumulation is increasing dramatically.**

- **Belly fat increases with a poor diet and physical inactivity.**

- **Belly fat has a number of negative effects on health.**

- **Belly fat is influenced by a variety of factors, including diet, inactivity, ethnicity, gender, age, stress, poor sleep and genes.**

- **Belly fat change can be assessed by measuring waist circumference, abdominal width and waist skinfold, and leg muscle mass change can be assessed by measuring girth circumference.**

You should now have an understanding of the difference between belly or visceral fat and subcutaneous fat, and of the dangers of carrying high levels of belly fat. You might even have identified factors in your own life that can lead to an increase of belly fat and will be able to estimate how much subcutaneous and belly fat you carry. Read on to learn the best ways to combat belly fat and create a healthier life.

Chapter 2
The effect of exercise on belly fat and health

Aerobic exercise can result in a loss in belly fat, however a lot of aerobic exercise has to be performed before results are seen. Similarly, carrying out 3 sessions of resistance exercise per week does not seem to reduce belly fat. In contrast, research has shown regular interval sprinting will reduce belly fat in far less time than other forms of exercise. In this chapter, you'll find a discussion of the results of published research articles that have examined the effect of aerobic and resistance exercise and interval sprinting on belly fat loss. There is also an examination of the possible mechanisms that are thought to contribute to the belly fat-reducing effect of interval sprinting and its effects on aerobic fitness, skeletal muscle mass and insulin resistance.

Aerobic exercise and belly fat

Traditionally, programs that use exercise to promote fat loss have consisted of participants engaging in a steady-state, moderate-intensity exercise such as walking, jogging or swimming for at least 45 minutes per session. The rationale for this is that individuals burn more fat as a fuel during moderate-intensity exercise and should lose more body fat as a result. Disappointingly, however, many studies have shown that this form of exercise leads to little total body fat loss unless the individual does very high volumes of aerobic exercise.[1] And while belly fat loss can occur after regular aerobic exercise, a lot of aerobic exercise has to be performed. For example, researchers at Duke University compared sedentary adults with adults who exercised at light or hard intensity. Results showed that the sedentary people gained about 9% of belly fat in 6 months, whereas adults who walked or jogged about 20 kilometres a week put on no belly fat. Those who jogged about 30 kilometres a week lost both belly and subcutaneous fat but their muscle mass was unchanged. A greater amount of belly fat (18%) was lost by overweight men and women who carried out a 14-week aerobic exercise program that involved exercising for 60-minute sessions 5 days per week. Again, their muscle mass remained unchanged.

A summary of results of the aerobic exercise studies in this area found that, to reduce belly fat, at least

30 minutes per day – and preferably up to 60 minutes per day – was needed for at least 14 weeks.[2] Thus, there is evidence to suggest that aerobic exercise for at least 45 minutes per day, 5 days per week, for 14 weeks can result in about an 18% decrease in belly fat without a change in muscle mass. As most people do not have the time or the motivation to engage in over 5 hours of exercise a week, there is need to find a form of exercise that results in a significant decrease in belly fat while maintaining or increasing muscle mass, and yet be time-efficient. Interval sprinting appears to be a form of exercise that meets these time constraints.

Resistance exercise and belly fat

Strength or resistance training – that is, exercising with weights – may also help reduce belly fat accumulation in some individuals. Researchers from the University of Pennsylvania monitored overweight and obese pre-menopausal women over a 2-year period. In comparison to women who performed no exercise, those women performing an hour of weight training twice a week decreased their total body fat by about 4%; however, while they did not record an increase in belly fat, the amount of belly fat was not reduced. Another 2 studies conducted with older men and women showed that 3 moderately hard weekly weight training bouts for 12 weeks resulted in little change in total body fat but a significant decrease in belly fat. A significant number of other studies, however, did not find any effect of resistance exercise on belly fat. A 2012 meta-analysis by one group of researchers reviewed the results of 35 well-controlled studies examining the effect of resistance exercise on belly fat and concluded that resistance training failed to induce significant reductions in belly fat.[3]

The weight training protocols used in these studies typically involved around 8 different exercises, with 8–10 repetitions, repeated 3 times each exercise. The individual exercises included upper arm, abdominals and leg muscles. This type of protocol was typically performed 2–3 times per week. During a typical 60-minute weight training session, the actual time spent lifting weights is about 8–10 minutes. Thus, it is likely that lifting weights at a moderate intensity for 8 minutes, 3 times per week will not result in significant decreases in body or belly fat.

What is interval sprinting?

Interval sprinting protocols typically involve repeated sprinting or hard exercise at near all-out intensity, followed by low-intensity exercise or rest. The length of the sprint period has varied from 6 seconds to 2 minutes, and the recovery period has ranged from 12 seconds to 4 minutes. Most researchers in this area have examined interval sprinting on a stationary cycle ergometer and have examined adolescents, young people, older individuals and patient groups consisting of cardiac rehabilitation, intermittent claudication, type 2 diabetes and obese children and adults. One of the most utilised protocols has been the Wingate test, which consists of 30 seconds of all-out sprint with a hard resistance. Subjects typically perform the Wingate test 4–6 times, with each sprint being separated by 4 minutes of recovery. Knowledge about changes to skeletal muscle from interval sprinting has been achieved mainly by using this protocol. However, the Wingate test is extremely hard and people have to be highly motivated to tolerate a lot of pain and discomfort. Consequently, the Wingate test is unsuitable for most overweight, sedentary individuals interested in losing belly fat.

Other, less intense interval sprinting protocols have also been applied. For example, we have used an 8-second cycle sprint followed by 12 seconds of low-intensity cycling for a period of 20 minutes. Thus, instead of 4–6 sprints per session, as used in Wingate studies, subjects using the 8-second/12-second protocol sprint 60 times at a lower exercise intensity for a total sprint of 8 minutes, with 12 minutes of low-intensity cycling. For this method, the total exercise time is 20 minutes, plus a 4-minute warm-up and 4-minute cool-down. Thus, one of the features of interval sprinting is it takes far less time than traditional aerobic exercise protocols, making it a time-efficient strategy by which to accrue health benefits.

Interval sprinting and belly fat

Direct measures, like magnetic resonance imaging (MRI), and indirect measures, like waist circumference, have been used to assess the effects of interval sprinting on belly fat. Mourier and colleagues showed a 48% decrease in belly fat, measured by MRI, after steady-state aerobic exercise 2 days per week and interval training 1 day a week for 8 weeks in middle-aged men and women.[4] Another study with older men, also using MRI, found that 8 weeks of aerobic interval training, which also involved hard exercise for 2 minutes and resting for 4 minutes, resulted in a 14% loss of belly fat.

Our research has used a shorter interval sprinting protocol with younger overweight people. In our first 2 studies with women, we used DEXA and waist circumference to assess belly fat change. DEXA does not directly assess belly fat but does measure a variable called central abdominal fat, which is highly related to belly fat. The first study we conducted lasted 15 weeks and our candidates did 20 minutes of interval sprinting at an 8-second/12-second ratio, 3 times per week.[5] They lost 2.6kg of total body fat (11%), which was accompanied by a significant decrease in central abdominal fat. In a second study, overweight women exercised for only 12 weeks using the same protocol.[6] They lost 9% of total body fat (2.5kg) and experienced a 6% decrease in central abdominal fat. In this study, waist circumference was reduced by 3.5cm after 6 weeks of interval sprinting. Waist circumference is highly related to central abdominal fat, which suggests that belly fat was significantly reduced after 6 weeks, or 6 hours, of interval sprinting. Women in this study also changed their diet in favour of a Mediterranean eating plan, which resulted in a 13% decrease in daily caloric intake.

In a third study, we examined a 12-week interval sprinting program on the belly fat of young overweight men.[7] In this study, we measured belly fat with a technique called computed tomography, which uses ionising radiation to locate the belly fat deep inside the abdomen. Males lost 9% of total body fat (2kg) and 17% of belly fat. They also lost 5% of subcutaneous abdominal fat. Similar to our studies with women, waist circumference was reduced by 3.5cm after 6 weeks of interval sprinting. In the male study, waist circumference was highly correlated with belly fat, suggesting that belly fat was significantly reduced after 6 weeks, or 6 hours, of interval sprinting. A summary of the results of studies examining the effects of aerobic exercise, resistance exercise and interval sprinting on belly fat reduction is shown in Table 3.

Because interval sprinting has only been studied relatively recently with subjects who are not athletes,

	Interval sprinting	**Aerobic exercise**	**Resistance exercise**
Range of total body fat loss	2-2.5kg	1-1.5kg	No change
Range of belly fat percentage loss	17-48% reduction	6-18% reduction	No change
Average waist circumference loss	3.5cm	2.0cm	No change
Average hours of exercise	12 hours	70 hours	36 hours

Table 3. A summary of the results of randomised controlled studies examining the effects of aerobic exercise, resistance exercise and interval sprinting on total and belly fat reduction.

Adapted from information found in studies by Boutcher et al., Ohkawara et al., and Ismail et al. [8]

there are fewer published research studies in this area. But it already looks like interval sprinting has resulted in far greater reductions of total body and belly fat than the other 2 exercise modalities in significantly less exercise time. It takes just 6 weeks of interval sprinting exercise to see a significant reduction in waist circumference, so we can conclude that the most effective form of exercise for reducing belly fat is interval sprinting.

Possible reasons interval sprinting leads to belly fat loss

The mechanisms underlying the interval sprinting-induced belly fat loss include increased exercise and post-exercise fat burning, increased muscle mass, decreased appetite after exercise, and reduced postprandial lipemia, which is when triglyceride levels in blood rise after eating. These levels can stay elevated for up to 18 hours.

Increased fat burning

Towards the end of an interval sprinting session that involves many repeat sprints, the exercising muscles start to run out of sugar, which, in the form of glucose and glycogen, is needed to create a high-energy compound called adenosine triphosphate (ATP), which provides the energy for muscular contraction. Towards the end of an interval sprinting session, it is thought that the ATP is mainly derived from intramuscular fat stores, the fat stored within the skeletal muscles. Together with subcutaneous and belly fat, these depots are an important source of fat. If we don't regularly burn up the fat accumulated inside our muscles, then the result is usually the development of insulin resistance and type 2 diabetes. When we deplete the fat stores inside the muscle by interval sprinting, however, the body is forced to replace them with fat stored elsewhere, such as in the belly and under the skin. This shuttling of fat from the belly to the skeletal muscle may also happen after exercise has stopped, as some of the hormones generated during interval sprinting appear to continue burning fat long after exercise. Because the fat stored in belly fat cells is more responsive to interval sprinting, we think that this shuttling of fat from the belly to the skeletal muscles contributes to long-term reduction of belly fat stores.

The ability of aerobic exercise to burn up extra energy after aerobic exercise has been extensively studied. A review of these studies concluded that a session of aerobic exercise lasting 40 minutes or more typically generated an increase in energy of about 13%. This is a negligible effect and is likely to make only a small contribution to overall fat loss. The fat-burning response after interval sprinting, however, has not been extensively examined. It is possible that the high blood catecholamine levels occurring during interval sprinting (see Figure 10, page 85) could induce fat burning long after exercise has stopped. This elevation may also happen because of the necessity to lower blood and muscle lactate – a chemical that accumulates during hard exercise – and to re-synthesise the depleted glycogen in the exercising muscles. The elevated growth hormone levels documented after a session of interval sprinting may also contribute to enhanced energy expenditure and fat burning.

Increased muscle mass

It has been estimated that an increase of 1kg of skeletal muscle has the capability to burn up about an extra 21 calories per day. In theory, this could amount to just under 3kg of body fat usage per year. Thus, retaining or increasing muscle mass is very important for health. Unfortunately, it is well documented that participating in aerobic exercise does not change muscle mass, while moderately hard resistance exercise may result in increased muscle mass in some people. A recent review concluded that weight-training programs carried out by middle-aged people resulted in an average increase of muscle mass of 1.2kg.[9] As can be seen in Table 5 (page 56), our 3 interval sprinting studies resulted in significant increases of leg and trunk muscle mass of 0.2kg and 0.3kg for women and 0.5kg and 0.7kg for men.[10] Another research group found a large increase in leg muscle mass of older women after they had carried out interval training for 16 weeks. These results are important, as muscle mass affects health and is typically reduced by ageing and when people go on a severe diet.

Decreased appetite

It is also possible that interval sprinting may result in suppressed appetite, which could contribute to belly fat loss. Studies on rats have shown that they eat less after they perform hard exercise. The mechanisms underlying this effect are not known, but hard exercise may reduce hunger by releasing hormones that decrease appetite. For example, corticotropin releasing factor, a powerful hormone that depresses appetite, has been shown to increase in rats and humans during hard running and swimming exercise. Although human studies have shown a large decrease in appetite after intensive aerobic exercise, this effect lasts only for a short time.

The effect of high-intensity sprinting on appetite suppression has been investigated by one study, which examined the effect of intensive exercise on the appetite of obese adolescents.[11] Appetite was assessed before and after a 6-week high-intensity exercise and diet intervention. The intensive exercise program increased the energy expenditure of the adolescents, however their appetites did not increase in line with their energy output. Why individuals do not eat more after hard, intensive exercise is unclear but animal studies have shown that appetite centres in the brain are affected by blood lactate levels. Lactate levels are increased in the blood when people do hard anaerobic exercise such as interval sprinting. Interestingly, in animals, injections of lactate have been shown to suppress appetite. Thus, it is feasible that the increased blood lactate levels brought about by interval sprinting may contribute to suppressed appetite in humans.

Decreased postprandial lipemia

Consuming saturated fat or fructose in 3 meals per day can result in elevated triglyceride (also called triacylglycerol) levels in the blood for up to 18 hours. This is called postprandial lipemia and is discussed in greater detail in Chapter 4. It has been discovered that people with high levels of fat in their blood after eating also tend to have greater belly fat stores. Impressively, just 1 bout of acute, moderately hard aerobic exercise lasting 40 minutes resulted in significantly lower fat in the blood after consumption of a high-fat meal even as long as 12 hours after exercise. Recently, we have shown that interval sprinting has a similar effect. Twenty minutes of interval sprinting at night reduced by about 20% the fat (triglycerides) in the blood of young women who ate a high-fat meal the next morning.[12] The mechanism underlying this effect is believed to be the ability of moderately hard exercise to increase an enzyme called lipoprotein lipase, which is located in the muscle capillaries. One of the major roles of lipoprotein lipase is to remove triglyceride from the blood in the circulation into the muscles that have been exercised. The increase in lipoprotein lipase found after exercise usually peaks after about 4–6 hours but stays elevated for up to 18 hours post exercise.

This effect of exercise on lipoprotein lipase may also play a critical role in the belly fat reduction found after interval sprinting. As discussed, the major hormones that induce fat release from belly fat cells are the catecholamines. Interval sprinting, in contrast to moderate aerobic exercise like walking, results in significantly greater blood levels of catecholamines. We have discovered that belly fat is far more sensitive to the effect of catecholamines than are the fat cells beneath the skin, so more fat is released from the belly fat cells during interval sprinting than from other fat stores. However, all belly fat that is released goes directly to the liver via the portal vein, where most of it is repackaged as triglyceride and secreted back into the circulation. So where does this fat in the form of triglyceride go? Although studies have not yet determined the destination, it is feasible that the increased triglyceride circulating in the blood, similar to the elevated triglyceride found after a high-fat meal, is shuttled into the skeletal muscle by the increased levels of lipoprotein lipase caused by exercise. This sequence of events is illustrated in Figure 4 (see page 48).

How much body and belly fat is it possible to lose after interval sprinting?

The amount of total body fat loss expected to happen after involvement in any exercise program can be assessed by estimating the energy cost of the exercise.

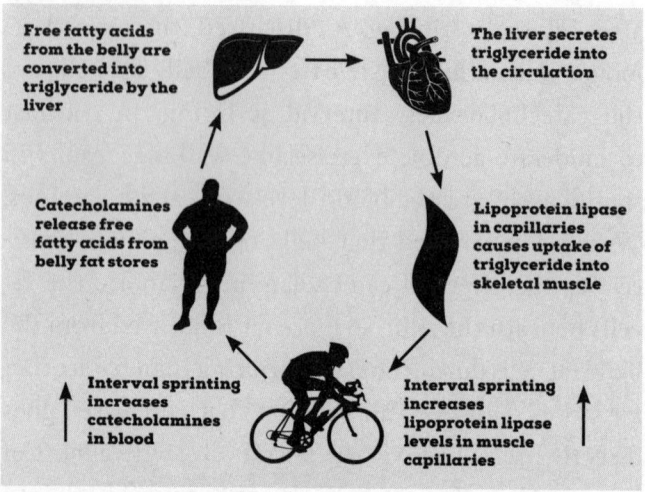

Figure 4. Interval sprinting may enable fatty acids to be transported from belly fat cells into the liver and then back into the circulation in the form of triglyceride, where they are shuttled into the skeletal muscles.

For example, the largest amount of fat the body of an untrained individual can burn during a bout of aerobic cycle exercise has been estimated to be around 0.6 gram per minute. Assuming an optimal fat metabolising rate of 0.6 gram per minute for one 60-minute session of cycling exercise would result in an energy usage equivalent of about 36 grams of fat. In optimal circumstances, a 12-week aerobic exercise program consisting of cycling 5 times a week for 60 minutes each session at a moderately hard exercise intensity could theoretically result in a fat mass loss of around 2.9kg, after adding the potential 13% more fat burning that may occur after the exercise has stopped. Over a year of exercise, fat loss could theoretically be around 12.6kg.

However, as mentioned previously, fat loss from aerobic exercise is usually much less than this amount because of a number of factors, such as compensatory eating and reduction in other forms of daily physical activity. Also, a range of individual, physiological and medical factors likes genes, fat-burning ability and thyroid dysfunction may impede fat loss in certain individuals.[13] In contrast, some people who exercise may lose much greater amounts of body fat, which most likely reflects the fact they've undertaken a starvation diet at the same time as they start their exercise program. Consequently, the most likely explanation for large increases or decreases in total fat mass after exercise is a change in diet. As we'll see in Chapter 4, starvation diets don't work for most people in the long term and are associated with a number of health problems. A reasonable amount of total body fat loss to expect after 15 weeks of interval sprinting is around 3.0kg.

The decrease in dangerous belly fat, however, is difficult to estimate, although it is known that belly fat is easier to lose than subcutaneous fat. For example, as mentioned earlier, in our previous study men lost 17% of their belly fat, 9% of their total subcutaneous fat and 5% of their subcutaneous abdominal fat.[14] Thus, percentage-wise, they lost 3 times more belly fat than abdominal fat after 12 weeks of interval sprinting. Similar to our study with women, waist circumference of these men was reduced by 3.5cm after 6 weeks of interval sprinting. Importantly, waist circumference was highly correlated with belly fat, suggesting that just 6 weeks of interval sprinting training, which involved eighteen 20-minute interval sprinting sessions – only a total of 6 hours of interval sprinting – produced a significant reduction in the amount of the individuals' belly fat.

The fitness, muscle mass and insulin-resistance response to aerobic, resistance and interval sprinting exercise

Reducing belly fat is a very important feature of interval sprinting, but there are other important adaptations that have big implications for health, including an increase in aerobic fitness and skeletal muscle mass and a decrease in insulin resistance.

Aerobic fitness

Aerobic fitness, typically called aerobic power by exercise physiologists, is very important for health. Maximum aerobic fitness is typically measured by getting subjects to exercise to exhaustion on a cycle or treadmill.

Gases are collected to assess the ability of an individual to deliver and use oxygen to the exercising muscles. Blair and colleagues found that aerobic fitness was strongly associated with early mortality.[15] Thus, fitter adults suffered fewer deaths from lifestyle diseases such as cancer, heart disease and stroke. These researchers showed that low aerobic fitness accounted for 16% of all deaths in a large group of American adults. This 16% contribution to total mortality is significantly larger than other risk factors, such as obesity, smoking, high cholesterol and diabetes. It has been well documented that being aerobically fit results in reduced risk for heart disease, metabolic disease, certain cancers and Alzheimer's disease. The good news is that interval sprinting significantly increases aerobic fitness even though the sprinting exercise is mostly anaerobic. We found that 15 weeks of interval sprinting resulted in a 26% increase in the aerobic fitness of young women, compared to a 19% increase in another group who completed 15 weeks of moderate aerobic exercise.[16] The interval sprinting consisted of 3 20-minute sessions per week, compared to 3 40-minute sessions of aerobic cycling exercise. In a second study with young overweight women, we found that 12 weeks of interval sprinting resulted in an 18% increase in aerobic fitness, while a 16% increase occurred in young overweight men.[17] Thus, a very important characteristic of interval sprinting is that it results in large increases in aerobic fitness. As interval sprinting is mostly anaerobic in nature, it also results in large increases in anaerobic fitness.

Skeletal muscle mass

Retention of skeletal muscle mass is very important when it comes to your health. For example, women who possess less muscle mass have greater incidence of osteoporosis. We typically lose a significant amount of our muscle mass as we age, and people who go on starvation diets generally lose significant muscle mass. As can be seen in Table 4 (page 53), women who went on a starvation diet, reducing their daily caloric intake by 50%, lost about 3kg of muscle over a 16-week period. Since it has been estimated that an increase of 1kg of skeletal muscle could use up just under 3kg of fat per year, any loss in muscle mass can result in a reduced incidence of fat loss, so retaining or increasing muscle mass is very important for health.

Unfortunately, even exercising does not stop the loss of muscle when dieting. When women performed either aerobic or resistance exercise while on a starvation diet, they still lost muscle mass but the loss was reduced by between 40% and 50%. It is well documented that participating in aerobic exercise does not change muscle mass, whereas moderately hard resistance exercise may result in increased muscle mass for some. As can be seen in Table 4 (see page 53), 3 interval sprinting studies showed significant increases of leg and trunk

Intervention	Weight loss	Fat-free mass loss/gain	Daily caloric decrease
LCD alone	-11.1 kg	-3.1 kg	50%
LCD with aerobic exercise	-11.4 kg	-1.5 kg	50%
LCD with resistance exercise	-11.6 kg	-1.98 kg	50%
ND with interval sprinting	-1.5 kg	+.6 kg	none
MD with interval sprinting	-1.9 kg	+.5 kg	13%
ND with interval sprinting	-1.5 kg	+1.2 kg	none

Table 4. A comparison of muscle mass loss with no dieting (ND), moderate dieting (MD) or low-calorie dieting (LCD) with or without aerobic, resistance and interval sprinting exercise.

Adapted from information in studies by Kuk et al., Trapp et al., Dunn et al. and Boutcher et al. [18]

muscle mass of 0.3kg and 0.4kg for women and 0.5kg and 0.7kg for men. Our study that examined interval sprinting and dieting is particularly interesting, as we asked overweight women to switch to a Mediterranean eating plan, which resulted in a daily caloric intake decrease of 13%. Despite eating slightly less every day, these women still significantly increased the amount of muscle in their legs (0.3kg) and trunk (0.3kg) and reduced their body fat by 2.6kg after 12 weeks of interval sprinting. These results suggest that combining healthy eating, such as the Mediterranean eating plan, with 12 weeks of interval sprinting may be the optimal way to lose belly fat and enhance muscle mass.

Insulin resistance

Insulin resistance is measured by assessing the amount of insulin and glucose in the blood. If these levels are high, it indicates that a person's tissues, especially the skeletal muscles and liver, are becoming resistant to the effects of insulin. Insulin, as you may recall, is released from the pancreas when we eat sugar. It enables the sugar in the blood to enter the tissues, to be used as energy by the cells or to be stored as glycogen for later use. Only insulin and exercise can remove sugar from the blood. Failure to reduce blood sugar levels over time is bad for health and typically leads to the development of type 2 diabetes. Participation in all forms of interval sprinting, aerobic exercise and resistance exercise typically decreases insulin resistance, and we found a large decrease in insulin resistance in 2 of our studies. The women who participated in the 12-week study reduced their incidence of insulin resistance by 31%, while those in the 15-week study experienced a reduction of 36%.[49, 50] In our study with overweight young women, their insulin resistance decreased dramatically after 6 weeks of interval sprinting. In comparison, aerobic exercise lasting greater than 12 weeks typically results in decreased insulin resistance of around 10%. Surprisingly, regular resistance exercise also decreases insulin resistance but the exercise has to be moderately hard.

Table 5 (page 56) was constructed by reviewing the results of articles that examined the maximum oxygen uptake, muscle mass and insulin-resistance reduction reponse to aerobic, resistance and interval training. Although fewer interval sprinting studies have been completed, interval sprinting has resulted in as big or bigger positive changes in maximum oxygen uptake, muscle mass and insulin-resistance than both aerobic and resistance exercise.

The typical amount of reduction of insulin resistance in study participants in randomised controlled studies lasting greater than 2 weeks was between 20% and 50%. We now think interval sprinting is especially suitable for individuals who suffer from type 2 diabetes and metabolic syndrome.

	Interval sprinting	**Aerobic exercise**	**Resistance exercise**
Maximum oxygen uptake increase	16–25%	12–20%	No change
Muscle mass increase	0.5–1.2kg	No change	0.5–1.2kg
Insulin-resistance reduction	20–50%	Around 12%	Around 10%
Average hours of exercise	12–15 hours	36–48 hours	36–48 hours

Table 5. A summary of the maximum oxygen uptake, muscle mass and insulin-resistance reduction repsonse to aerobic, resistance and interval training in randomised control trials lasting at least 12 weeks.

Interval sprinting and special populations

There are now over 50 articles published in scientific literature examining different aspect of interval training. Surprisingly, a number of these articles have examined the effects of interval training on the health of special populations, including heart disease, intermittent claudication and diabetic patients, depressed individuals, older people, postmenopausal women and post-pregnant women. Interval training protocols in these studies have varied but most research groups have used longer interval exercise at a less than all-out intensity for 2 minutes, followed by low-intensity exercise or rest for 4 minutes. Thus, although cycling for a 2-minute bout cannot be classed as sprinting, the exercise was still performed at high intensity and followed by a rest. Although more research needs to be done in this area, the preliminary results are promising.

Heart disease patients

The heart is the organ that pumps blood to all body tissues; if it stops pumping, death quickly follows. There are a number of heart diseases but 2 major ones are coronary artery disease and chronic heart disease. Coronary artery disease occurs when the arteries that provide blood to the heart don't work properly; if they become blocked, blood cannot get to the heart. Blocked arteries in the heart can be caused by smoking, high cholesterol, hypertension, type 2 diabetes and inherited genes. Chronic heart disease is a condition where the heart does not pump normally and is usually caused by a weak cardiac muscle or faulty heart valves. Heart disease is the major cause of death in most Westernised countries.

A number of studies have investigated the effect of interval training on patients possessing coronary heart disease and chronic heart failure. A series of studies carried out on coronary artery bypass patients by one research team in the 1990s showed that, compared to control groups, their physical performance significantly improved after a program of interval training.[19] Another team examined the effect of interval exercise on stent function following heart surgery. Results showed that high-intensity interval exercise improved stent function, increased aerobic fitness and reduced inflammation.[20] A different study compared the effects of aerobic interval training and moderate continuous aerobic training on aerobic fitness and quality of life after coronary artery bypass grafting.[21] Four weeks of interval and continuous aerobic exercise showed a significant increase in aerobic fitness of all participants; however, 6 months later, the interval group had greater aerobic fitness than the continuous exercise group. Interval training protocols in these studies involved cycling at less than all-out intensity for 2 minutes, immediately followed by rest for 4 minutes.

With regard to chronic heart disease patients, one study found that 16 weeks of high-intensity interval training enhanced functional capacity and quality of life.[22] Another study compared the effect of moderate aerobic and high-intensity exercise on cardiovascular function in heart failure patients: aerobic fitness was increased more with aerobic interval training and was associated with greater improvements in left ventricular function.[23] A different study also showed that high-intensity interval exercise was better than moderate continuous aerobic exercise for increasing aerobic fitness in coronary artery patients.[24] Collectively, research examining interval exercise and coronary artery disease and chronic heart failure has shown that interval training increases aerobic fitness in far less time than conventional moderate aerobic exercise. Quality of life was also consistently improved, as were a number of indicators of heart function. An overview of this area has been provided by Ernst.[25]

Chronic obstructive pulmonary disease patients

Chronic obstructive pulmonary disease affects breathing and is characterised by chronic bronchitis or emphysema, which results in narrowed airways in the lungs. Chronic obstructive pulmonary disease is typically caused by smoking, which inflames the lungs. In the US it is the third leading cause of death and it has been calculated to cost over US$42 billion in increased health care and lost productivity. Estimates suggest that chronic obstructive pulmonary disease will become the fourth leading worldwide cause of death by 2030.

Patients with this disease usually have trouble performing aerobic exercise and typically have an overall poor quality of life. When performing continuous aerobic exercise, chronic obstructive pulmonary disease patients typically experience breathing discomfort and have to stop for a rest. As exercising and resting is the basis of interval training, it appears that this form of exercise is suitable for chronic obstructive pulmonary disease patients. A 12-week study compared interval with aerobic exercise and found that patients with chronic obstructive pulmonary disease significantly improved their exercise tolerance after interval exercise.[26] Continuous aerobic exercise also improved exercise tolerance but involved twice as much exercise time. After both interval and aerobic exercise, quality of life was significantly improved. These results have been replicated in a number of studies. In another study, researchers showed that both interval exercise and continuous moderate aerobic exercise resulted in positive changes to muscle function, however interval training caused fewer training problems.[27] Interval training protocols in these studies typically involved a less than all-out intensity cycling for 30 seconds, immediately followed by a rest for 30 seconds.

Overall, research examining interval exercise and chronic obstructive pulmonary disease has shown that interval sprinting increases aerobic fitness in less time than moderate aerobic exercise. Quality of life was also consistently improved. Importantly, interval training caused fewer training problems, such as shortness of breath and breathing discomfort. Because interval training allows chronic obstructive pulmonary disease patients to tolerate harder intensity exercise for longer periods of time with less breathing and leg discomfort, it appears to be superior to other training modalities.[28]

Metabolic syndrome and diabetic patients

Metabolic syndrome is a condition distinguished by having a lot of belly fat, high blood pressure, insulin resistance and bad blood-lipid profiles. It is a precursor to type 2 diabetes and is typically an outcome of an unhealthy diet and being sedentary. Incidence of type 2 diabetes has substantially increased during the last 50 years in a similar fashion to rates of obesity: in 2010 there were about 285 million people possessing metabolic syndrome compared to about 30 million in 1985. Worryingly, the World Health Organization has estimated that by 2025, 50% of the world's type 2 diabetics will be people of Asian descent.

Long-term complications caused by type 2 diabetes are heart disease, stroke, retinopathy, kidney disease and nerve degeneration. Type 1 diabetes is a form of diabetes that results from the inability of beta cells in the pancreas to produce insulin. The degradation of the beta cells is usually brought about by our immune systems. In Western countries, type 1 diabetes comprises about 10% of the total diabetic population. Most people who develop type 1 diabetes are usually of average weight and healthy in comparison with those who develop type 2 diabetes.

Aerobic exercise has been shown to be beneficial for reducing symptoms of metabolic syndrome and type 2 diabetes. The effects of interval training, however, have been less examined but initial results are promising. For instance, one study placed 32 metabolic syndrome patients on a 16-week program of interval training and found that many health risk factors were reversed.[29] Another examined the effects of resistance and interval exercise training on skeletal muscle function in people with type 2 diabetes.[30] They found that 10 weeks of resistance and interval training in unfit type 2 diabetic patients resulted in improvements in muscle function and blood pressure. Interval training protocols in these studies involved less than all-out intensity cycling for 2 minutes, immediately followed by resting for 4 minutes. A further study investigated the effects of low-volume interval sprinting – 10 cycle bouts of 60 seconds with 60-second rest periods for 20 minutes – on glucose regulation and skeletal muscle metabolic capacity.[31] Results showed that low-volume interval sprinting rapidly improved glucose control and induced skeletal muscle adaptations that were beneficial for the health of patients with type 2 diabetes.

The effects of a single 10-second sprint on glucose levels of exercising type 1 diabetics have also been investigated. It is well established that moderate intensity aerobic exercise increases the risk of hypoglycemia (low blood-sugar levels) after exercise in those with type 1 diabetes. Therefore, the study investigated whether a short, 10-second cycle sprint would prevent the rapid fall in blood sugar levels typically associated with moderate aerobic exercise in individuals possessing type 1 diabetes.[32] Their results indicated that for individuals possessing type 1 diabetes who participated in moderate aerobic exercise, a 10-second maximum sprint at the end of aerobic exercise prevented a fall in blood-sugar levels. Another study assessed whether 30 minutes of interval sprinting resulted in less lowering of blood-sugar levels compared to 30 minutes of continuous aerobic exercise.[33] The decline in blood sugar levels was less with interval sprinting compared with aerobic exercise in people with type 1 diabetes.

Collectively, research examining interval exercise and metabolic diseases such as type 2 diabetes has shown that interval training consistently increases insulin sensitivity and reverses a number of risk factors. An overview of this area has been provided by Kessler and colleagues.[34]

Depressed individuals

Depression is a long-term mood disorder and is usually defined as having continuous unhappiness and reduced enjoyment of everyday life for greater than 2 weeks. It has been estimated that about 1 in 7 people in Westernised countries are clinically depressed. People who experience depression typically have a range of health problems, such as cardiovascular disease, headaches, back pain, anxiety attacks and poor-quality sleep. Depressed individuals exhibit chronic increased levels of cortisol, which causes increased belly fat accumulation.

In 2008, investigators from Amsterdam found that depressed people had twice the risk of gaining belly fat over a 5-year period compared to people without depression. These authors suggested that storing fat in the belly puts depressed people at much greater risk for cardiovascular disease and diabetes. It has been shown that depressed individuals have much greater incidence of heart disease and diabetes.

Interestingly, these investigators found no association between depression and obesity. This finding suggests that, despite being of normal weight, depressed people had elevated levels of belly fat. Another study examining women found similar results. The study assessed depression levels and belly fat of middle-aged African-American and Caucasian women and found a strong relationship between depression and belly fat; no association between depression levels and subcutaneous fat was found. Although it is not clear how depression causes an increase in belly fat, it is possible that depression triggers the accumulation of belly fat by increasing the production of cortisol and inflammatory compounds.

Can depression be reduced by exercise? Yes. Research has shown that all kinds of moderately vigorous exercise tend to alleviate clinical depression. For depression reduction, moderately vigorous exercise such as fast walking, jogging and strength training compared to easy exercise produced the best results. Depression has been shown to change in weeks, however longer exercise programs seem to produce greater reductions in depression levels. Whether or not the positive effect of exercise on depression is related to decreased belly fat is unknown. That longer, moderately vigorous exercise tends to alleviate clinical depression more may indicate that these kinds of exercise programs result in a greater reduction of belly fat.

The effect of interval sprinting on depression has not been examined, however, given the large reductions in belly fat occurring after interval sprinting and the connection between belly fat and depression, its potential appears to be significant. Interval sprinting may be suitable for depressed patients because it can be fun, can be performed in a group, is time-efficient and has been shown to reduce belly fat.

Intermittent claudication patients

Intermittent claudication is skeletal muscle pain experienced as aching, cramping and numbness, which usually occurs in the calf muscles when walking and is only relieved by resting. Intermittent claudication is due to peripheral artery disease brought about by blockages of the arteries of the leg. People who smoke, have high blood pressure or possess type 2 diabetes have a greater incidence of intermittent claudication. Men over 50 have the highest incidence of intermittent claudication, and it affects around 5% of people in Western populations.

A number of studies have shown that regular aerobic exercise can improve intermittent claudication symptoms. Patients typically walk for 5 minutes, rest for 5 minutes, and then repeat this pattern for 20–30 minutes. However, one study found that high-intensity training at 80% of maximum oxygen uptake was more effective than an identical volume of low-intensity training for improving aerobic fitness in patients with intermittent claudication.[35] The high-intensity training patients carried out 2 minutes of speed walking on a treadmill, followed by 3-minute sit-down resting periods. This was performed 8 times. Another study conducted a high-intensity rehabilitation program with intermittent claudication patients that lasted 12 weeks. Patients walked on a treadmill for 6 minutes at a speed that brought about ischaemia and maximum claudication pain. When patients reached this level, they stopped walking and rested for 3 minutes. Patients performed this protocol 6 times per session. Results showed that those patients who successfully completed the 6 sessions showed the greatest decrease in claudication symptoms. The authors concluded that, as no adverse events were experienced, patients with intermittent claudication can safely tolerate high-intensity exercise programs.[36]

Obese and overweight adults and children

Obesity is a condition in which body and belly fat accumulation negatively affects health. It increases an individual's chances of heart disease, type 2 diabetes, sleep apnoea and certain cancer types. Obese individuals also have a reduced life expectancy. People are classified as obese when their BMI exceeds 30. Obesity is typically caused by genetic influences, excessive food energy intake and being sedentary, although some people can become obese because of endocrine disorders and certain medications. There has been a dramatic increase in overweight and obesity over the last 50 years in both developed and developing countries.

Does participation in aerobic exercise significantly reduce body fat of obese and overweight individuals? The answer is no; regular aerobic exercise only results in a minor loss in total body fat. It results in a greater loss of belly fat if individuals are prepared to exercise for at least 1 hour, 5 times per week. The good news is that participation in interval sprinting does significantly impact on body fat if individuals are prepared to exercise for 1 hour per week. We have shown that interval sprinting results in a significant reduction of total body fat and belly fat of overweight – where BMI equals 28 – women and men.[37] Other researchers studied the effects of a 12-week, high-intensity exercise program on obese older men and women and found a significant reduction in belly fat, while subjects in a moderate-intensity group showed no decrease in belly fat.[38] Similarly, another study found that interval training significantly reduced belly fat in older men and women.[39] Importantly, they found that reductions in belly fat were strongly related to reductions in insulin resistance – the greater the reduction in belly fat, the greater the improvement in insulin sensitivity.

With regard to childhood obesity, one study compared the effects of high-intensity exercise and a multi-treatment strategy on a number of cardiovascular risk factors in obese adolescents.[40] One group performed aerobic interval training twice per week for 12 weeks: 4 minutes of hard uphill running on a treadmill followed by 4 minutes of rest. Another group undertook a multi-disciplinary approach over 12 months, including dietary changes, moderate exercise and psychological advice twice a month. The results indicated that high-intensity exercise brought about a greater reduction in cardiovascular risk factors than the multi-treatment strategy.

Overall, research examining the effects of high-intensity exercise and interval sprinting exercise on the obese and overweight has shown that this kind of exercise decreases body fat to a greater extent than continuous aerobic exercise. Belly or visceral fat has been shown to be reduced by interval sprint training in far less time than by aerobic exercise. Because interval training, especially on the stationary bike, is easily performed by obese adults and children, and because it results in more subcutaneous and belly fat loss, it appears to be superior to other kinds of training.[41]

Postmenopausal women

Premenopausal women are typically younger than 46 and tend to have less belly fat than men, as they store their fat in their legs, hips and on the back of their arms. This differing pattern of fat storage for women and men is mainly an outcome of the hormone oestrogen. As women go through menopause in their late 40s and early 50s, however, oestrogen production stops or slows down, resulting in increased belly fat accumulation. Scientists have suggested that the reduction in oestrogen is also accompanied by an increase in the stress hormone cortisol which, as mentioned previously, helps increase belly fat. Thus, women older than 46 tend to have greater increases in belly fat than males. Women in their late 40s can find their waistlines increasing even if they don't gain much weight, as increasing belly fat forces the abdominal wall outwards.

Importantly, diet is relatively ineffective at reducing the belly fat stores of postmenopausal women. In one study, postmenopausal women only lost belly fat when exercise, in the form of walking, was added to a diet. Interval training, however, has been shown to result in greater belly fat reductions in postmenopausal women. The previously mentioned study of middle-aged men and women showed a 48% decrease in belly fat, measured by MRI, with an 18% decrease in subcutaneous fat after steady-state aerobic exercise 2 days per week and interval training 1 day a week for 8 weeks.[42] Another study carried out on 32 middle-aged metabolic syndrome men and women over 16 weeks involved interval training 3 times per week. Aerobic fitness of participants was enhanced by 26%, whereas body weight was decreased by 2.3kg.[43]

Overall, research examining the effect of interval exercise on postmenopausal women's health has shown that interval training or sprinting increases aerobic fitness in less time than moderate aerobic exercise. Body fat also decreases to a greater extent after interval training interventions compared to continuous aerobic exercise. Belly or visceral fat has also been shown to be reduced by interval training in far less time than aerobic exercise.

Pregnancy and interval sprinting

Many women increase their food intake excessively when pregnant, and while there are general guidelines to help women understand how much weight gain is appropriate during pregnancy, there are no specific guides regarding the amount of fat that should include. Weight gain during pregnancy is influenced by the baby's weight and the mother's increase in blood volume and body fat. Some fat stores are increased during pregnancy to enhance breast feeding but excessive fat gain increases a number of health risks for mother and baby. Unfortunately, a significant amount of women increase their belly fat stores during pregnancy. Although many women think they have to 'eat for 2' when pregnant, only a small number of extra calories are needed. While pregnant women should not be encouraged to diet to lose weight, as this may harm the health of the growing baby, a healthy diet and regular physically activity are important for the long-term health of both mother and baby.

But what about after pregnancy? Given that many women will retain their increased belly fat stores after giving birth, and that interval sprinting has been shown to decrease belly fat in non-pregnant women, it follows that interval sprinting may be the optimal exercise for reducing these unwanted belly fat stores. Research studies, however, are needed to confirm this relationship.

With regard to conception, no studies have investigated the effect of interval training on conception rates. Some research has been done with aerobic exercise and it seems that really hard exercise, like marathon training, is detrimental, while moderate exercise –

3 45-minute sessions of aerobic exercise per week for example – is beneficial for conception. So where would interval sprinting fit in? Interval sprinting is performed at a harder intensity but is much shorter than a 45-minute bout of aerobic exercise. In our studies with women aged between 18 and 30, we did not have any reports of menstrual irregularity after training 3 times per week for 12 or 15 weeks. With regard to belly fat and conception, it has been shown that those women possessing elevated belly fat stores have a reduced rate of conception. As interval sprinting has been shown to reduce belly fat in women, it is feasible that interval sprinting may enhance conception rates, but research into this area is required.

*

In the research described above, all subjects or patients were medically screened before participating in high-intensity interval training. It is important that you seek medical advice on the possible positive or negative effects of interval training on your health before beginning an interval sprinting regime. The potential interaction between any medication you might be taking and interval training should also be estimated. For example, if you have heart disease and are taking some form of beta blocker, you will not be able to elevate your heart rate to the recommended level during exercise.

An accredited exercise physiologist (EP) qualified to give advice on exercise and beneficial life changes, such as diet, stress-management and sleep quality enhancement, together with a physician who is supportive of lifestyle change strategies is the ideal team to help as you embark on an interval training program. They will be able to advise you on what form of exercise to do, how long each session should last and how many times per week you should exercise and at what intensity. You can find an exercise physiologist near you by visiting www.essa.org.au.

If you are just interested in improving your fitness and health, then most types of continuous, steady-state exercise will be effective. If, however, you want to lose belly fat and improve your insulin sensitivity, as well as improve your aerobic and anaerobic fitness and increase muscle mass, then interval sprinting is the best option. See Chapter 3 for more information on incorporating the interval sprinting program in your life.

*

The points highlighted above outline the way we should be exercising if we want to lose belly fat. It's important to remember the following:

- Aerobic exercise can result in a decrease in belly fat but people have to exercise at a moderately hard intensity for at least 5 hours per week.

- Resistance exercise does not seem to decrease belly fat in most people.

- Interval sprinting has resulted in an 17% decrease in belly fat when males exercised for 1 hour per week for 12 weeks.

- We're not sure how interval exercise works on belly fat, but it's likely that increased fat burning during and after exercise and a possible decrease in appetite are the main factors.

- Interval training has been used successfully in a number of special populations, such as heart disease and type 2 diabetes patients.

Chapter 3
The interval sprinting belly fat loss program

Now you're familiar with how belly fat affects your health and the positive effects interval sprinting can have on the amount of belly fat you carry, let's outline a 8-second sprint/12-second recovery interval sprinting program, the benefits such a program offers, equipment you'll need and how to begin training.

What happens to heart rate and hormones during interval sprinting?

Heart rate

There are a number of acute responses to interval sprinting, but 3 that are important for belly fat loss are heart rate, blood lactate and fat-burning hormones. Your heart-rate response depends on what type of interval

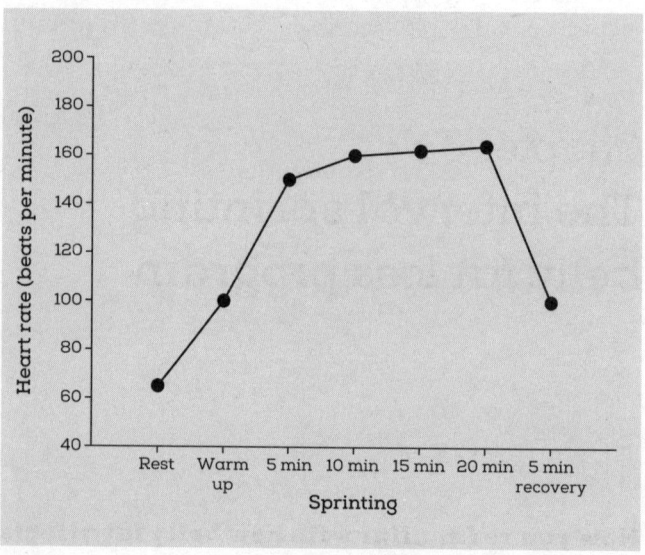

Figure 5. The heart-rate response of young adults to 1 session of interval sprinting consisting of an 8-second sprint and 12 seconds of easy pedalling for 20 minutes.

sprinting protocol you undertake, but typically it is significantly elevated during interval sprinting exercise and declines slightly during the recovery between sprints. For example, peak heart rates during the hard Wingate test typically exceed 170 beats per minute during a 30-second all-out cycle sprint, with the average heart rate across the 30-second sprint being 150 beats per minute. Studies have found a smaller heart-rate response for an interval sprinting protocol consisting of 10 6-second sprints interspersed with a 30-second recovery.[1] Heart rate increased to 142 beats per minute after the first sprint and then increased to 173 beats per minute following sprint 10. Heart-rate response to the 8-second/12-second program typically averages around 150 beats per minute after 5 minutes of interval sprinting, which then increases to 160 beats per minute for young adults after 15 minutes of exercise.[2] As can be seen in Figure 5 (page 76), the heart rates of young adults gradually increase during the 20 minutes of 8-second/12-second interval sprinting. In the 8-second/12-second program, there is typically a small heart rate decrease of around 3–5 beats per minute during each recovery period.

So we know that heart-rate response to interval sprinting varies depending on your age. In young adults, heart rate typically averages around 150 beats per minute after 5 minutes of interval sprinting, which then increases to 160 beats per minute after 20 minutes of exercise. For middle-aged adults, optimal heart-rate response is generally lower, around 140 beats per minute after 5 minutes of interval sprinting, increasing to 150 beats per minute after 20 minutes of exercise.

Measuring heart rate

Heart rate during exercise and recovery can be measured manually or by a heart-rate monitor. The best place to measure heart rate during exercise or exercise

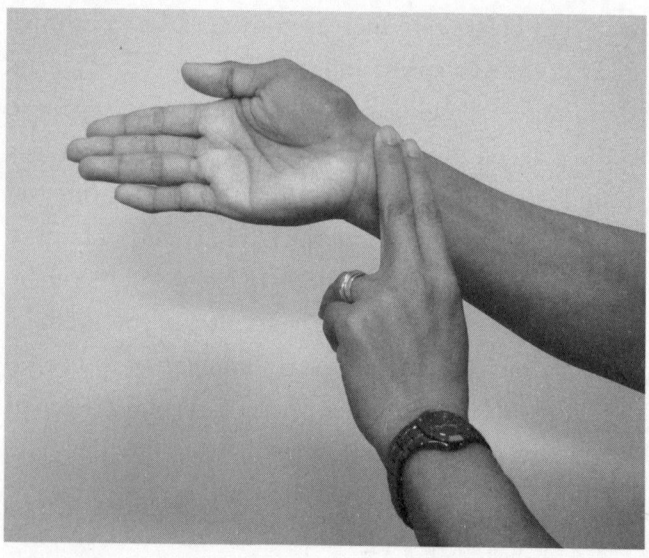

Figure 6. Locating the radial pulse at the base of the wrist.

recovery using the manual or palpation method is at the radial artery, located in the wrist. The fingers should be used to locate a pulse rather than the thumb.

To locate the radial pulse on your wrist, position the index and middle fingers on the opposite wrist, approximately 1.5cm on the inside of the wrist, below the index finger (see Figure 6, above). When the pulse is found, count the number of beats for 1 minute. The per-minute rate can also be calculated by counting for 10 seconds and multiplying by 6.

A heart-rate monitor is much easier and gives a much more accurate reading of your heart rate than using the

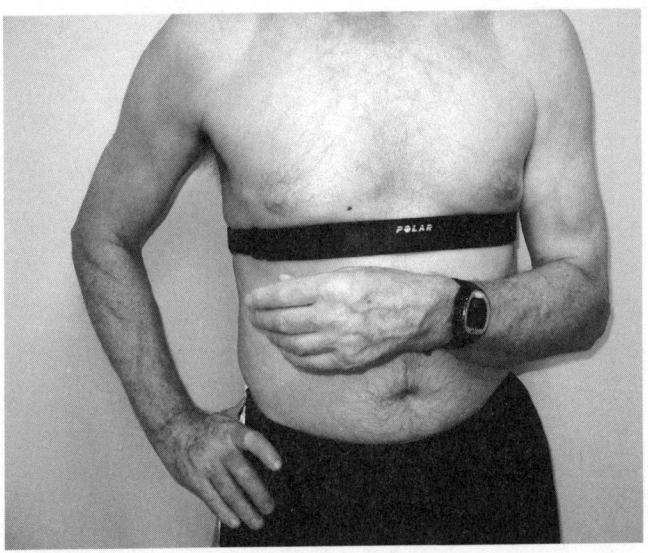

Figure 7. Assessing heart rate by using a heart-rate monitor.

finger palpitation method. There are numerous heart rate smartphone apps available for iPhones and Android devices that can measure heart rate. Using a heart-rate monitor, as pictured in Figure 7 (above), is also useful when you want to record your heart rates so you can examine them later. Such monitors also allow you to download your records to a computer.

Rating of perceived exertion

Exercise physiologists measure how hard people feel they are working during exercise by using a rating of

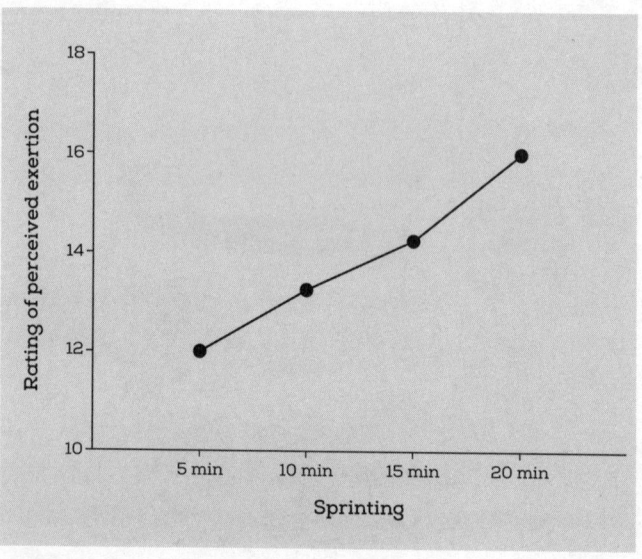

Figure 8. The rating of perceived exertion response of young adults to 1 session of interval sprinting consisting of an 8-second sprint and 12 seconds of easy pedalling for 20 minutes.

perceived exertion scale (see Appendix D, page 206). When exercising, people are asked to answer the question 'How hard are you working?' by indicating their perceived effort level on a scale that ranges from 6 to 20.[3] When performing lower-intensity interval sprinting such as the 8-second sprint/12-second recovery program, the rating of perceived exertion is usually around 12 and increases to just over 15 by the end of the session. This can be seen in Figure 8 (above).

When performing aerobic exercise, the rating is typically equivalent to about one-tenth of the exercise heart rate. Thus, a rating of 16 would typically accompany a heart rate of 160 beats per minute for young adults in their 20s. For aerobic exercise, if you increase the intensity of exercise as you get fitter, your rating of perceived exertion typically stays the same. We have shown that this is not the case with interval sprinting.[4]

With interval sprinting exercise, the rating is typically equivalent to about one-eleventh of the exercising heart rate, so a rating of 14 would typically accompany a heart rate of 150 beats per minute for young adults. As people get fitter with repeated interval sprinting, they will typically increase pedal rate and resistance. After interval training, however, instead of staying the same, the rating of perceived exertion tends to go up. This is probably because the greater force developed by skeletal muscles needed to cope with higher pedal resistance loads on the bike causes higher exertional perceptions. Thus, as force production increases, the greater amount of signalling received by the brain's sensory centres could be the reason why the rating of perceived exertion goes up after interval sprinting training.

Blood lactate levels

Lactate is a chemical that accumulates in the blood when an individual does anaerobic exercise, which is performed at a higher intensity than aerobic exercise. Anaerobic exercise uses energy systems that do not require oxygen, relying mainly on glycolysis to release energy into the muscles, and is typically brought into action when performing brief, high-intensity bouts of exercise continuously, as with interval sprinting. Heavy use of the glycolytic pathways during this kind of exercise results in enhanced acidity in the exercising muscles – lactate – which then spills into the blood.

Exercise physiologists measure blood lactate levels to gauge how much energy is being derived from the glycolytic pathways. Blood lactate levels are low while at rest but can significantly increase during anaerobic exercise. For example, blood lactate levels during the high-intensity Wingate test protocols are typically 6–10 times higher than those at rest. Lactate levels gradually increase during longer, lower-intensity interval sprinting protocols such as the 8-second/12-second for 20 minutes protocol and are usually between 2 and 4 times greater than those at rest after 5 minutes of interval sprinting for both trained cyclists and untrained women who took part in our study (see Figure 9, page 83). Lactate levels were about 5 times greater than those at rest after 15 minutes of interval sprinting. Thus, lactate levels immediately increase at the start of interval sprinting and continue to slowly increase throughout the exercise session. Despite increasing lactate levels during sprinting exercise, it appears that

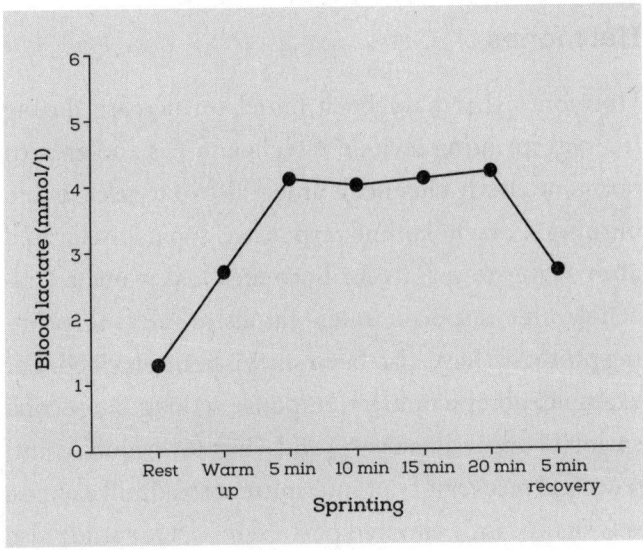

Figure 9. Blood lactate response of young adults to 1 session of interval sprinting consisting of an 8-second sprint and 12 seconds of easy pedalling for 20 minutes.

fat transport is also increased. For example, a 20-minute session of 8-second/12-second sprinting resulted in elevated levels of glycerol, reflecting increased release of fatty acids into the blood.[5]

Blood lactate levels gradually increase during interval sprinting such as the 8-second/12-second for 20 minutes protocol and are usually 3–4 times greater than resting values at the end of a 20-minute session.

Hormones

Hormones that have been found to increase during interval sprinting include catecholamines and growth hormone, both chemicals integral to fat release and burning. Catecholamine response is typically elevated after Wingate sprints for both men and women. Catecholamine response to less-intensive interval sprinting protocols have also been shown to be elevated. For example, norepinephrine response to long (24-second sprint/36-second recovery) and short (6-second sprint/9-second recovery) bout intermittent treadmill exercise was significantly elevated post exercise. Our study also found significantly elevated epinephrine and norepinephrine levels after 20 minutes of interval sprinting cycle exercise – 8-second/12-second and 24-second/36-second programs – in trained and untrained young women (see Figure 10, page 85).[6] Another study examined the catecholamine response of 12 males who performed 10 6-second cycle sprints with a 30-second recovery between sprints. Compared to baseline, plasma epinephrine increased 6.3 times, whereas norepinephrine increased 14.5 times at the end of sprinting.[7] This large catecholamine response to interval sprinting is in contrast to moderate, steady-state aerobic exercise which typically brings about small increases in epinephrine and norepinephrine. The interval sprinting catecholamine response is an important finding, as catecholamines are

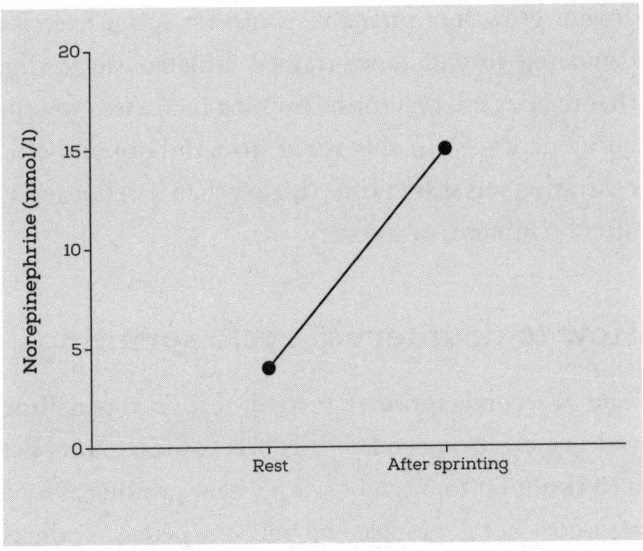

Figure 10. The norepinephrine response of young adults to 1 session of interval sprinting consisting of an 8-second sprint and 12 seconds of easy pedalling for 20 minutes.

the major drivers of fat release from both belly and muscle depots.

Growth hormone also induces fat burning by coaxing fat cells to release fat. Growth hormone has been shown to increase during high-intensity exercise. With regard to interval sprinting, one study investigated the growth-hormone response to 30-second treadmill sprinting.[8] Male and female athletes displayed a marked growth-hormone response, and there was a greater growth-hormone response for sprint exercise compared to endurance-trained athletes, suggesting that regular interval sprint training increases growth-hormone levels. In this study, growth-hormone concentration was still 10 times higher than baseline levels after 60 minutes of recovery.

How to do interval cycle sprinting

The 8-second sprint/12-second recovery pedalling cadence is recommended. It is best to wear shorts but a tracksuit bottom can be worn when sprinting as long as it does not get tangled up with the pedals. Trainers are suitable for footwear, and when cycling inside, it is a good idea to have a towel handy to remove excess sweat. In average temperature conditions (20–24°C), 20 minutes of interval sprinting typically results in a sweat loss of around 0.3kg. You can measure your sweat loss during exercise by simply measuring your nude weight before and immediately after an interval sprinting session: if you weigh 70kg nude before sprinting and 69.7kg nude after the session then you would have lost 0.3kg of sweat. Sweat loss is usually significantly greater when exercising in hot, humid conditions. Information concerning choosing and setting up the bike, selecting a suitable pedal rate and resistance, and determining your optimal heart rate and rating of perceived exertion are included below.

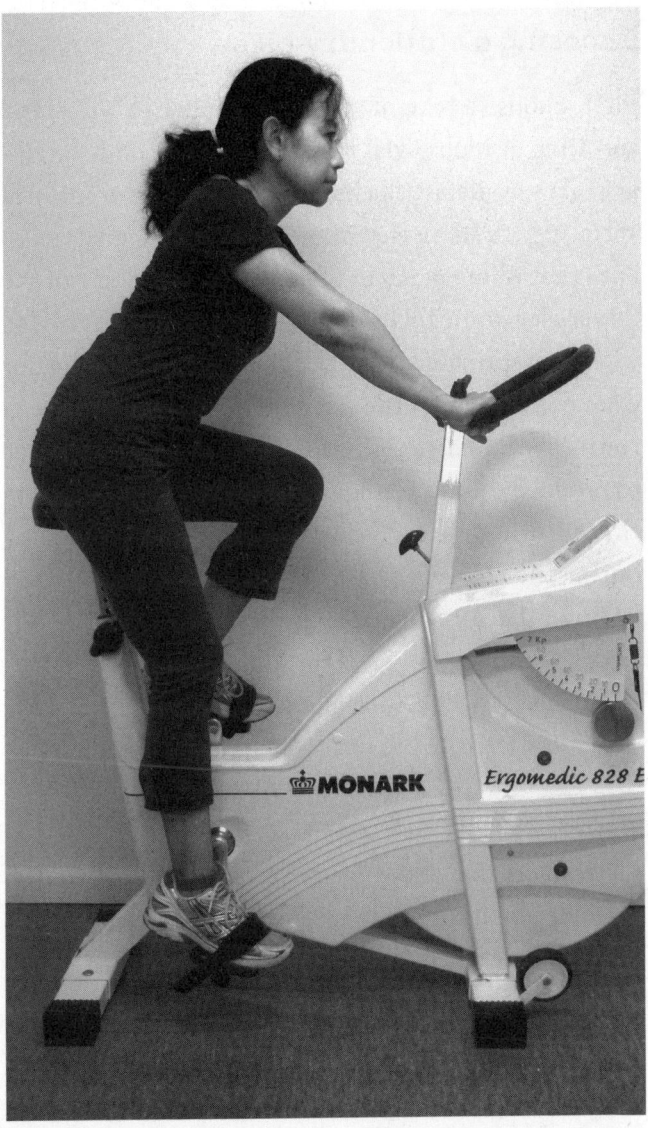

Figure 11. The set-up for performing interval sprinting on a stationary bike.

Choosing a stationary bike

First, choose a bike of sufficient quality to withstand sprinting at high pedal rates. Of the range of stationary bikes available, the most suitable ones for interval sprinting are those that allow you to set a pedal resistance that is independent of power output. Some of the newer electronic bikes do not allow you to do this, so when you sprint against a pedal resistance of 1.0kg, for example, instead of the resistance staying the same in the recovery phase, the bike will increase the resistance to produce the same amount of work generated during the sprinting phase. What should be easy pedalling during the recovery phase becomes hard exercise, and having a hard recovery phase will prevent the body from oxidising the waste products produced during sprinting. It will also make the workout excessively demanding, tiring you out more quickly.

How to set up the bike

First, adjust the saddle height so when you're sitting on the bike you have about a 5% bend at the knee. Adjust the handle bars so your hands rest on top of them. Make sure that the pedals have foot grips. The correct set-up for sprinting is shown in Figure 11 (page 87).

Choosing the pedal rate and resistance

We know that the production of catecholamines during bike interval sprinting is brought about by moving the legs quickly: cycling fast is more important than cycling hard. Your pedal rate will be influenced by a range of factors, such as your fitness, age, health, leg muscle mass and height. It is best to start with a comfortable pedal rate and then increase it if your rating of perceived exertion is less than 12 and your heart rate is low for your age.

The pedal rate is more important than the load. This means a woman with no health issues could start on a 0.5kg resistance and sprint at 100 revolutions per minute. Fitter or stronger women may require a heavier load, say 1.0kg, and sprint at more than 100 revolutions a minute, while a smaller, older female who is unfit might need to start at a pedal resistance of 0.5kg and a pedal rate of 90 revolutions per minute. A man with no health issues should start at 1.0kg resistance and a pedal rate of 100+ a minute, while fitter, stronger men should be able to sprint at a pedal rate of 115 revolutions a minute.

Stationary bikes have a number of different ways of varying pedal resistance. Increasing pedal resistance is similar to cycling up a hill: the steeper the hill, the greater the pedal resistance. Stationary bikes typically control pedal resistance by either tightening a band around the wheel or by slowing the wheel with magnets. Most bikes will quantify pedal resistance in kilograms or pounds. On the Monark bike made in Sweden, for example, tightening the strap on the wheel from 0.5kg to 1.0kg when pedalling at 100 revolutions per minute will double the power output, which is how much power you are generating when cycling and is typically measured in watts. Watts are calculated by multiplying the pedal rate by the pedal resistance. Thus, cycling at 100 revolutions per minute at a resistance of 1.0kg is equivalent to a power output of 100 watts. If all this sounds too technical, don't worry. In their first session, most people should try to pedal at a rate of 100 revolutions per minute with a resistance of 0.5kg.

You will have to increase the load and pedal rate as you enhance your fitness with training. For the first week of training, if you're unfit, you should try 10 minutes of interval sprinting and then see how you feel at the end of the session and when you wake up the next morning. If everything is fine, then you should increase the exercise time to 15 minutes during week 2. By week 3, most people should be able to complete the full 20 minutes of interval sprinting. After 2–3 weeks, you will probably find that your sprint pedal rate is too low. If your rating of perceived exertion is low (12 or less) then you should increase your pedal rate. Try an increase of 5 revolutions per minute, for example, from 90 to 95, and see how your rating of perceived exertion and heart-rate change.

Heart rate and rating of perceived exertion during interval sprinting

Monitoring your heart rate is important, although, working out your optimal interval sprinting heart rate is tricky. Typically, exercise physiologists determine exercise heart rates firstly by calculating an individual's maximum exercise heart rate which they do by continually increasing the power output on a bike until the exercising person reaches exhaustion and their heart rate will not increase any further. Maximum heart rates typically, but not always, reduce with age; a person in their twenties may have a maximum heart rate of 200 beats per minute, whereas a person aged 60 years may have one of 160 beats per minute. For interval sprinting, the optimal heart rate is typically around 75–80% of a person's true maximum heart rate: for a young person an exercise heart rate averaging 150 beats per minute would be appropriate, while for a 70-year-old person an exercise heart rate averaging 113 beats per minute may be optimal.

Unfortunately, most people do not know their maximum heart rate. It can be estimated by using the Karvonen formula, which simply calculates the required heart rate by assuming maximum heart rate can be estimated by subtracting a person's age from 220. Thus, a person aged 20 would have an estimated maximum heart rate of 200 beats per minute: 220 − 20 = 200. A person aged 60 would have one of 160 beats per minute: 220 − 60 = 160. However, young people can have a maximum heart rate of 160 beats per minute and older people, especially if they are fit, of over 200 beats per minute.

If you do not know your true maximum heart rate, the best strategy is to use a trial-by-error approach. For example, an unfit but healthy 20-year-old male could start interval sprinting by using a pedal rate of 100 revolutions per minute at a resistance of 0.5kg. If his true maximum heart rate was 200 beats per minute, then his exercise heart rate should be around 150 beats per minute. As discussed below, the rating of perceived exertion for a heart rate of 150 when interval sprinting is around 14 − somewhat hard to hard. If the rating of perceived exertion was 17 − very hard − then it is likely that the true maximum heart rate of this individual is lower than 200 beats per minute, therefore a heart rate of 150 beats per minute when exercising would likely be too much. Optimal target heart rates are around 150–160 beats per minute for most people in their 20s, 130–140 beats per minute for most people in their 40s, and 120–130 beats per minute for most people in their 60s.

Heart rate will continue to increase during a 20-minute session of interval sprinting. Thus, at the start of exercising you do not want your heart rate to be too high, for example, 160 beats per minute, as it will end up around 170 beats per minute. Heart rate is also affected by heat, which means exercising in warm, humid conditions will result in much higher heart rates, as the heart has to work harder to cool you by shunting blood to your skin.

It is also important to measure your heart rate at the end of the 4-minute cool-down period. If your heart rate got up to 160 beats per minute it should get down below 100 beats per minute by the end of the 4-minute cool-down. As you get fitter, your cool-down heart rate should decrease more quickly.

How to do your first session of interval sprinting

Before starting a high-intensity interval training program you should be medically screened. This is especially important if you are older, have any risk factors, have any diseases or are on medication. Being screened means the possible positive or negative effects of interval training on you are being assessed by a physician. If you live in Australia, an accredited exercise physiologist will also be able to give you more information and advice for this kind of exercise.

Make sure you have decided on a suitable pedal rate – 90–130 revolutions per minute for most untrained people – and pedal resistance – between 0.5kg and 1.5kg. Perform a 4-minute warm-up using continuous cycling at 60–90 revolutions per minute with a resistance of 0.5kg. This should result in a rating of perceived exertion of around 11. If your rating of perceived exertion is higher – say, 13 – then you should decrease the resistance and pedal rate. If you are not using LifeSprint music (see page 97) then you need to time the warm-up, sprinting, recovery and cool-down phases. You can download apps for iPhones and Android devices that allow you to create your own interval sprinting program. The LifeSprint music will prompt you to get ready for the sprint through a 3, 2, 1 countdown, and the sprint component of the music is fast whereas the recovery is slow. Therefore, you have to learn to sprint during the 8-second fast music and slow your pedalling rate during the 12 seconds of slow music. If you are timing yourself, increase your pedal rate 3 seconds before the actual sprint.

When sprinting, the pedal rate displayed on your bike will always lag behind the real pedal rate, although some bikes do not display or record pedal rate. By the end of the 8-second sprint, the bike should have caught up and be displaying the real pedal rate. It's important that you learn the feeling of your targeted pedal rate so it can be performed throughout the 8-second sprint, without relying on the bike to tell you what your rate is.

When sprinting, pushing and pulling with your legs is very important. When you push down on the pedal, you activate the quadriceps muscle, located on your upper thigh, and when you pull the pedal up with your legs, you activate the hamstrings, located underneath your thigh. It is much easier to cycle at high pedal rates if you use this push/pull technique. If you only use a push action, which is typical for beginners, then it makes the sprinting feel much harder. Using the push/pull technique involves more leg muscle mass and should produce more fat burning. It is advisable to push back slightly on the handlebars with your arms to stabilise your pelvis to prevent rocking and bouncing. This avoids possible soreness after interval sprinting exercise.

What does interval sprinting feel like?

For most people, the first couple of sprints of a session feel quite hard, but when they have established a rhythm it gets easier. Most people will not start breathing heavily until after about 5 minutes of sprinting; this is also the time they typically start sweating. We think this is because this form of exercise starts to deplete the short-term energy supplies in the exercising muscles after about 5 minutes, meaning the body has to switch to sugar stores inside the muscle to provide the fuel for sprinting. Towards the end of the sprinting session, we think fat stored inside the muscle is also used, and it continues to be used during the recovery period. Breathing is likely to become heavier.

As fat burning is more likely to occur in the latter stages of the session, you should keep working at the correct intensity right throughout the 20 minutes. Towards the end of the 20-minute session your legs should be feeling slightly tired. After 20 minutes of interval sprinting, however, you should feel energised rather than exhausted.

It is important to perform the 4-minute cool-down so that the heart rate can return to lower levels before you get off the bike. A pedal rate and resistance lower than your warm-up – for example, 50 revolutions per minute at 0.5kg – should see your heart rate go below 100 beats per minute by the end of the cool-down. If your heart rate does not decrease quickly, then change your maximum pedal rate and resistance to 50 revolutions per minute at 0.25kg. Jumping off the bike immediately after sprinting is unadvisable, as it may cause blood pooling and fainting.

What is the best time of day to do interval sprinting?

The best time of day for interval sprinting is early in the morning, before breakfast. If you can do it without eating any food, we believe it will result in increased fat burning. If you can only exercise at lunchtime, try to stop eating for 2–3 hours before exercise and drink only water or green tea for as long as possible before your session. Exercising at night is probably the second-best option, as long as you can ingest your evening meal at least 2 hours before your session. For example, eating at 5 pm and exercising at 7 pm will give time for the insulin in your blood to subside.

Remember, insulin is elevated after eating sugar and protein and encourages fat storage rather than fat burning, so try to drink only water or green tea for as long as possible after exercise. Ingestion of sugar or protein before or after exercise will immediately result in an increase in blood insulin levels that will impede fat burning. The advantage of exercising at night is that you can avoid eating for at least 8 hours after exercising because you are asleep, which will allow the body to burn more fat, assuming you only drink water or green tea after exercise.

Music for interval sprinting

Performing interval sprinting to music makes it much more enjoyable, and while interval sprinting can be performed without music, attempting to time each sprint and recovery session tends to make the experience tedious. Music specifically developed for interval sprinting called LifeSprints is available on iTunes.

Methods of interval sprinting

There are a number of different methods for performing interval sprinting, including the following:

Sprint cycling

Cycling on a stationary bike is probably the optimal form of interval sprinting, as it is non-weight-bearing and thus less stressful on ankles, knees and hips. Most research examining the effects of interval sprinting has used the stationary bike, and there are a number of unique aspects of the stationary bike that other forms of exercise do not possess. For instance, the bike allows people to complete a significant amount of sprinting without getting exhausted. If a person uses the 8-second/12-second protocol and cycles at a pedal rate of 125 revolutions per minute during sprinting, then they would have sprinted 6.0 kilometres during the 20 minutes of exercise. If their rate was 85 revolutions per minute during each rest period, they would have pedalled an additional 6.1 kilometres, making a total cycling distance of 12.1 kilometres in a 20-minute session. The 8-second sprint protocol involves 60 sprints, resulting in a total of 1006 pedal revolutions for 8 minutes of sprinting during the 20-minute session. Thus, the optimal interval sprinting protocol would be to sprint 6 kilometres of distance using about 1000 pedal revolutions.

	Light	Moderate	Hard
Pedal rate sprinting	90rpm	115rpm	125rpm
Pedal rate recovery	50rpm	75rpm	85rpm
Pedal resistance	0.5kg	1kg	1.5kg
Distance sprinted	4.3km	5.5km	6.0km
Distance recovery	3.6km	5.4km	6.1km
Total distance	7.9km	10.9km	12.1km
Total sprint cycles	720	920	1000
Average sprint power output per 8-second sprint	45 watts	115 watts	188 watts

Table 6. Example pedal rates and distance cycled for a 8-second sprint/12-second recovery protocol for 20 minutes at light, moderate and hard exercise intensities (rpm = revolutions per minute).

Table 6 (on page 99) shows the pedal rates and distance cycled for low, moderate and hard interval sprinting cycle workouts.

These 1000 pedal revolutions place significant overload on the major leg muscles, such as the hamstrings, quadriceps and gastrocnemius. This stress placed on the legs is the likely explanation for the significant increase in muscle mass that we found in our 3 studies (see Table 4, page 53). Women increased their leg muscle mass by 0.2kg whereas men increased theirs by 0.5kg.

However, in all 3 studies the biggest increase in muscle mass was found in the core muscle area, which includes the rectus abdominis, external and internal obliques, and transverse abdominis. These muscles are isometrically contracted during sprinting to provide a platform from which to turn over the legs quickly. Isometric muscle contraction occurs when a muscle is contracted but does not change its length. In our 3 studies, both women and men had significant increases in these core muscles, with 0.4kg for the women and 0.7kg for the men. This increase in muscle mass after cycle interval sprinting is very important because, as mentioned earlier, it has been estimated that for each 1kg increase in muscle mass there's an increase of daily energy burning of about 21 calories. If this muscle mass increase was maintained for 1 year, it would likely increase energy expenditure by about 7665 kilocalories, which would be equal to burning about 1kg of fat.

The workout that the leg muscles receive is likely to be the major reason why all studies that have examined cycle interval sprinting and glucose metabolism have shown that it reduces insulin resistance. This finding has major implications for the prevention of type 2 diabetes, which has been shown to be a disease of the legs and liver.

Sprint rowing

Rowing on a stationary rowing machine is a good form of interval sprinting exercise. This exercise is also non-weight-bearing but involves more muscles than cycling, as it uses the upper body. As the limbs do not move as quickly as in cycling, however, it is not clear how sprint rowing will affect belly fat. Young adults performing interval sprint rowing in our laboratory have easily got their heart rates up to similar levels as those generated on the stationary bike, so it is likely that sprint rowing induces significant elevations in catecholamines. Studies measuring the catecholamine response to sprint rowing, however, need to be performed.

Sprint walking

Sprint walking can utilise fast-twitch muscle fibres but probably not to the same extent as cycling. Nevertheless, it is a reasonable form of exercise for those who like to walk, but it is very difficult to get a young adult's heart rate over 130 beats per minute when sprint walking. Therefore, it is unlikely that sprint walking will result in significant reductions in belly fat.

Sprint stair climbing

Sprint stair climbing is a good form of interval sprinting as it is possible to get your heart rate over 130 beats per minute. The advantages of stair climbing are that it avoids pollution and traffic, and is cheap and time-efficient. Stair walking is a low-impact exercise, although descending is harder on joints.

The recommended posture is to keep a straight back, to avoid extending the knees and to place all of the foot on the step. You should ensure the staircase you choose is well ventilated and lit, has an even surface and offers good personal safety. We recommend you wear cross trainers rather than running shoes. The net energy cost in calories of stair climbing when walking has been estimated to be about 0.15 calories per 20cm step for a 70kg male. This is about 1 calorie for 7 steps. The optimal stair climbing walking rate has been estimated to be 90 steps per minute, so for 270 steps – 3 minutes of climbing – the energy cost is just below 40 calories. Coming down the stairs burns about a third of the energy as going up. Going up and down for 1000 steps per day would use up about 143 calories.

Stair climbing programs typically take about 12 minutes a day and are usually split into 3 4-minute sessions. Interval sprint stair climbing could include a 8-second stair climb and then a 1-minute toning exercise with the use of body weight and rubber bands. Other exercises could include push-ups against the wall and sit-ups.

Sprint running

Sprint running is another form of interval sprinting exercise. It is possible for experienced runners to do it on a treadmill, however this is a high-risk exercise. Because a treadmill is not able to accelerate and decelerate quickly enough for the 8-second/12-second protocol, you have to set the treadmill to sprinting speed and then jump off the treadmill while holding on to the side bars for the 12-second recovery phase before jumping back on to sprint.

Sounds too dangerous? Then try it on a running track. Sprint for 8 seconds and then easy jog for 12 seconds. Do this continuously around the track. If you don't have a track, you can try sprint running on a flat, grassy surface. Map out a triangle and sprint for 8 seconds on one side of the triangle then easy jog for 12 seconds on the other 2 sides. This is probably the hardest type of interval sprinting; for some people, it will place too much stress on their ankle and hip joints.

Sprint arm ergometry

Upper-body interval sprinting training involves rapid movement of the arms. No research to date has investigated the effect of upper-body interval sprinting on muscle adaptations or clinical markers like blood and muscle lactate. It is likely, however, that this form of exercise will bring about changes that are similar to lower-body interval sprinting, although these changes will be to a lesser extent. Moving the arms rapidly can be achieved by a number of exercise modalities, although the most efficient is the stationary arm ergometer, a piece of equipment similar to a stationary cycle.

Sprint boxing
Boxing, especially with a partner, is another form of upper-body interval sprinting exercise. You can do this by yourself if you have access to a punching bag. Your partner can also hold a foam impact pillow while you punch continuously for 8 seconds. During the recovery phase, you can shadow-box slowly for 12 seconds – for example, by slow ducking and weaving. Heart rates during this form of exercise can easily get up to 150 beats per minute for young adults; thus, boxing may result in reduced belly fat, but, as mentioned, the ability of methods other than cycling to reduce belly fat is undetermined.

Sprint skipping
Skipping rope is a good form of interval sprinting exercise that you can do by yourself or with a partner. You will need a skipping rope, a suitable surface and good-quality footwear. Sprint skip for 8 seconds and then easy jog on the spot for 12 seconds. Heart rates during

this form of exercise also can easily get up to 150 beats per minute for young adults.

Sprint swimming
Interval sprinting can be done in a swimming pool or in the ocean. A major limitation is timing the sprints or listening to sprint music. It would be possible with waterproof headphones, but counting the seconds as you sprint and recover is also an option. An example would be to sprint using freestyle for 8 seconds and then switch to easy breaststroke for a 12-second recovery period. It is difficult for non-athletes to get their heart rates up to 150 beats per minute while swimming, therefore it is unlikely that sprint swimming will result in a significant increase in catecholamines and, consequently, a reduction in belly fat.

Interval sprinting circuits
Interval sprinting circuit training is an excellent form of exercise that you can do by yourself, with a partner or in a group. Choose a combination of interval sprinting exercises from those listed above – for example, a good whole-body workout could include 5 minutes of boxing, 5 minutes of sprint skipping, 5 minutes of sprint rowing and 5 minutes of sprint cycling.

If you have time, it is possible to extend the 20-minute session by adding a resistance exercise between each sprinting exercise. For example, an interval sprinting circuit could include 5 minutes of boxing, 5 minutes of skipping rope, 5 minutes of rowing and 5 minutes of cycling. In between the sprinting bouts you could do 30 seconds of resistance exercises, such as push-ups, dips, crunches, biceps curls, lunges and so forth.

Monitoring your progress

To monitor your progress you need to record a certain amount of information. This information could include:

- heart-rate response during sprinting exercise
- heart-rate response during the cool-down
- pedal rate during bike sprinting exercise
- pedal resistance during bike sprinting exercise
- weight and/or body fat change
- waist circumference change
- abdominal width change
- waist skinfold site change
- lower- and upper-leg circumference change
- rating of perceived exertion during exercise
- aerobic fitness change, as assessed by a submaximal fitness test

Heart rate, pedal rate and pedal resistance have been previously described in this chapter, whereas body composition was outlined in chapter 2 (pages 34–74). Rating of perceived exertion is an easy but effective way of monitoring exercise intensity and has been used to prescribe exercise intensity in a variety of sporting activities and clinical settings. A rating of perceived exertion chart is typically used to measure people's perception of how hard they are exercising (see Appendix D, page 206).

Aerobic fitness change can be estimated by a submaximal fitness test (see Appendix B, page 202). Equipment required for this test is a stationary bike, a heart-rate monitor and a rating of perceived exertion scale. The test lasts only about 10 minutes with a 4-minute cool-down and can be performed every month to assess exercise heart-rate change. Three bike protocols for unfit, moderate and high fitness individuals are described on pages 110–111. All that is required is for you to perform the exercise protocol as described, and to record your heart rate and rating of perceived exertion at the end of each exercise stage. As can be seen, this submaximal test involves a 4-minute warm-up, an easy 3-minute cycling stage, a medium-hard 3-minute cycling stage and a moderately hard 3-minute cycling stage. The test should not be too tiring and it is important that your exercise heart rate does not go too high.

After you have finished the test, you should have your resting and exercise heart rates recorded, together with your rating of perceived exertion at the 3 stages. You can then plot these data on the graph included in Appendix C (page 204). You should see your heart rates increase during the 3 stages after the warm-up. If you are nervous and consequently have a high resting heart rate, your heart rate for stage 1 and 2 may be similar. When people get accustomed to the test, however, they typically get a consistent rise in their heart rate across the 3 stages.

Analysing the heart-rate response to submaximal exercise after 3 interval training studies conducted in our laboratory, we found that a decrease in the average heart rate by 1 beat at stages 2 and 3 equalled an increase in aerobic fitness of about 1%. Thus, after doing interval sprinting for 6 weeks, if the average heart rate at stages 2 and 3 was lowered by 4 beats per minute, the increase in aerobic fitness would be about 4%. Your heart rate will continue to decrease and you will get fitter if you either increase your pedal rate or resistance over the following weeks of exercise. For example, an average decrease in heart rate of 10 beats per minute for stages 2 and 3 equates to an increase of aerobic fitness of about 10%, and a decrease of 20 beats per minute about 20%, and so on.

The lowered heart rate during exercise reflects adaptations in the heart, the muscles and the blood;

it is not possible to have an increase in aerobic fitness without a lowering of heart rate at the same bike power outputs. A monitoring form to record all this information is included in Appendix F (page 210). You can copy the form and record this information every week for 6 weeks. Other information can be recorded on the weekly record form located in Appendix G (page 212).

On the following pages are examples of a morning, lunchtime and evening interval sprinting weekly program, performed at light, moderate and hard interval sprinting intensities. You should choose the method and exercise intensity that is best for you. You might also choose to exercise 2 mornings per week and once at lunchtime or in the evening.

What about exercising on the other days? It is likely that performing more interval sprinting exercise, either by increasing the length of each session, say, from 20 minutes to 30 minutes, or by including more sessions, such as adding 20 minutes of interval sprinting on a Sunday, will result in greater adaptations, such as reduced belly fat, increased aerobic fitness, decreased insulin resistance and increased leg and trunk muscle mass.

A morning workout (light)

	Before sprinting	Time of day: 6–8am	Pedal rate & resistance	Information recorded
Mon	Drink water or green tea	20 minutes of LifeSprints	90rpm at 0.5kg, 50rpm recovery	Weight and fat, exercise heart rate and RPE
Wed	Drink water or green tea	20 minutes of LifeSprints	90rpm at 0.5kg, 50rpm recovery	Exercise heart rate and RPE
Fri	Drink water or green tea	20 minutes of LifeSprints	90rpm at 0.5kg, 50rpm recovery	Exercise heart rate and RPE

A lunchtime workout (moderate)

	Before sprinting	Time of day: 12–2pm	Pedal rate & resistance	Information recorded
Mon	Fast for 2–3 hours and drink water or green tea	20 minutes of LifeSprints	115rpm at 1.0kg, 75rpm recovery	Weight and fat, exercise heart rate and RPE
Wed	Fast for 2–3 hours and drink water or green tea	20 minutes of LifeSprints	115rpm at 1.0kg, 75rpm recovery	Exercise heart rate and RPE
Fri	Fast for 2–3 hours and drink water or green tea	20 minutes of LifeSprints	115rpm at 1.0kg, 75rpm recovery	Exercise heart rate and RPE

An evening workout (hard)

	Before sprinting	**Time of day: 6-8pm**	**Pedal rate & resistance**	**Information recorded**
Mon	Fast for 2-3 hours after evening meal and drink water or green tea	20 minutes of LifeSprints	125rpm at 1.5kg, 85rpm recovery	Weight and fat, exercise heart rate land RPE
Wed	Fast for 2-3 hours after evening meal and drink water or green tea	20 minutes of LifeSprints	125rpm at 1.5kg, 85rpm recovery	Exercise heart rate and RPE
Fri	Fast for 2-3 hours after evening meal and drink water or green tea	20 minutes of LifeSprints	125rpm at 1.5kg, 85rpm recovery	Exercise heart rate and RPE

This chapter has described interval sprinting techniques and modalities. The key points to remember are:

- For best results, it's important to perform interval sprinting correctly by determining your optimal pedal rate and pedal resistance.

- **Interval sprinting can be performed successfully by a number of patient groups, provided they consult their GP and/or an exercise physiologist prior to beginning their program.**

- **It is important to monitor your interval sprinting performance and the health changes that are likely to occur with regular interval sprinting, so you can measure the amount of belly fat you lose.**

Now that you know how to choose the right equipment for interval sprinting and how to use it to get the most benefit from your program, let's look at adopting an eating plan that enhances your exercise program and helps you lose belly fat.

Chapter 4
Dieting, nutrients and belly fat

Why we have we become overweight

The last 50 years have brought an excessive abundance of high-energy processed food and a significant decrease in physical activity to our lives. Fat-inducing factors of the modern diet include increased consumption of sugar, high levels of saturated fat, increased use of unhealthy vegetable oils and inadequate consumption of fibre and the healthy fats found in foods such as olive oil, fish oils, avocado and coconut. Our bodies are very good at storing fat and poor at burning it up because for most of our evolutionary history we have never been faced with an abundance of food, and unfortunately modern processed foods tend to put the body into fat-storage mode as opposed to encouraging cells to burn fat. We're also moving less, because most of us sit down all day at our computers. Even our children don't move as much as they used to, thanks to a decrease in the amount of physical activity they engage in both at school and as recreation. As discussed in Chapter 5, increased levels of daily stress and reduced quality of sleep also affect fat gain.

To counteract these negative factors of modern living, we need to adapt a healthy eating regimen. The healthiest way of eating is based on consuming lots of fruit and vegetables and little processed food, a diet commonly known as the Mediterranean eating plan.

Our hunter-gatherer genetic legacy

The agricultural revolution occurred some 10,000 years ago, but human evolution began some 2.6 million years earlier, in the Paleolithic period.[1] This means we still carry a relatively unchanged ancient genome. Although we live in the 21st century, from a genetic perspective we are Paleolithic people. When hunter-gatherers adopted a diet based on grain, their health quickly degenerated, and this decline in health is prevalent today as lifestyle diseases continue to dominate Westernised and developing nations. We eat highly processed synthetic foods with up to 3 times less fibre, half as much polyunsaturated and monunsaturated fats, 4 times less fish, 60–70% more

How's your diet?

Use this questionnaire to assess your general diet and find out what changes you might need to make to help reduce the amount of belly fat you carry. Answer the questions below with regard to your typical eating patterns by filling in a score between 1 and 4 for each question and then sum your total.

1 = Not at all   2 = Sometimes
3 = Fairly regularly   4 = All the time

1. I eat junk food every day

2. I drink at least 1 soft drink every day

3. I eat sugary food such as cakes and sweets daily

4. I eat fried food every day

5. I eat pieces of fruit every day*

6. I eat servings of vegetables everyday*

TOTAL

* Reverse the scoring for questions 5 and 6:
4 = Not at all   3 = Sometimes
2 = Fairly regularly   1 = All the time

Interpreting your score:
6–9 points: low levels of processed food
10–12 points: moderately low levels of processed food
13–18 points: moderately high levels of processed food
19–24 points: high levels of processed food

saturated fat, 3 times more protein and up to 5 times more salt and sugar. Our problem is that our DNA has evolved in an environment of food scarcity, yet today we are immersed in an overabundance of inexpensive, processed, unhealthy food. Over centuries, our bodies have become very good at storing fat and until recently had never faced the problem of being overweight. Modern humans typically eat an excess of high-energy processed food and are unable to use up these extra fat stores.

The problem with modern processed foods

Sugar

Weight-inducing factors of the modern diet include increased consumption of sugars in general, and of fructose in particular. Fructose is a simple sugar that does not cause a high rise in blood sugar, so it was once recommended as a substitute for sucrose. While the body needs small amounts of fructose, too much overwhelms our liver. In developed countries, fructose now makes up a significant part of what we consume: it comprises about 10% of the average Western diet. When we eat excessive fructose, the liver's ability to metabolise it is diminished. Overwhelmed with fructose, the liver converts this sugar to fat and distributes the fat, in the form of triglyceride, into the circulation. Fruit and vegetables have small amounts of fructose, but food manufacturers also add lots of fructose to a wide range of foods. Much of this added fructose comes in the form of high-fructose corn syrup, which is very inexpensive. The problem is that fructose does not satisfy our appetite – in fact, fructose makes us feel hungry. Food manufacturers know that when they add fructose to a food, people eat a lot more of it. Consequently, excess fructose consumption is associated with fat gain.

Almost all packaged foods have some added sugar. In some countries you can check for added fructose by examining the labels of packaged foods; however, many countries do not differentiate between the different types of sugars on their labelling. Be particularly wary of soft drinks, as they are usually full of fructose, and even fruit juice usually has a lot of fructose – minus the healthy nutrients of whole fruit. All soft drinks should be eliminated from your eating plan and fruit juice consumed sparingly. As an example, a cup of chopped tomatoes has about 2.5 grams of fructose, a can of regular soft drink about 20 grams, and a super-size cola about 60 grams.

Fat

The second dangerous aspect of the modern diet is our tendency to eat the wrong kinds of fats. Consume healthy, monounsaturated fats and you will boost your body's fat-burning ability, but eat unhealthy, saturated or polyunsaturated fats and you will likely gain body fat.

Saturated fat is a hard fat and is contained in butter and meat. A US study conducted on men and women aged 55–75 years tried to determine if eating saturated fat contributed to belly fat accumulation. Subjects kept a food diary and underwent magnetic resonance imaging (MRI) to assess their belly fat. Results showed that those who ate the greatest amount of saturated fat also possessed the largest belly fat stores. Men and women who consumed more than 30% of their calories in the form of saturated fat had high levels of belly fat, so it's reasonable to expect that consuming lots of saturated fat in your diet increases the risk for accumulation of belly fat.

Vegetable oils are also troublesome, as they are full of polyunsaturated fatty acids that go rancid quickly. During preparation for the market these oils are typically heated and have solvents added and can also be exposed to air and sunlight. This processing destroys their nutritional value and also creates oxidants, which are dangerous for health. Canola, corn, safflower, soy and sunflower oils are among the most highly refined polyunsaturated oils. Also, polyunsaturated oils have been shown to slow down the thyroid gland and thus encourage fat gain. You should not heat any vegetable oil. Use coconut oil (a saturated fat) but don't heat to a temperature higher than 160°C. Coconut oil is full of saturated medium-chain fatty acids. It is unusual among saturated fats because studies have shown that natural coconut oil encourages fat burning, prevents certain diseases prevention and has anti-ageing properties. The medium-chain fatty acids in coconut oil go straight to the liver, rather than into the circulation, where they influence enzyme activity and induce fat burning. In contrast, long-chain fatty acids are typically stored as body fat. Coconut oil is also antibacterial and is very good for the skin. Coconut oil can be used for stir-fries, however the best way to stir-fry is to use no oil at all. Coconut butter is also an excellent substitute for butter and margarine. You can buy coconut oil in health stores, and there are numerous websites with recipes using coconut oil.[2]

Olive oil is another excellent fat that has proven health benefits. Your olive oil should be as fresh as possible, stored in the fridge, and kept away from sunlight. Buy small bottles and change them every 3–4 weeks. Make sure to buy local so that transit time is reduced.

Don't forget about fruits with high antioxidants, like avocado and papaya. Avocado has more fat than any other fruit, and, like olive oil, it is mainly in the form of healthy monounsaturated fat. Avocados are versatile and can be eaten as a snack, as a dip, added to a spicy pasta sauce or sliced on top of grilled chicken breast. They should be eaten raw.

Finally, omega-3 polyunsaturated fatty acids found primarily in oily fish have proven health benefits. Interestingly, it has been estimated that the great majority of people eating processed food diets are omega-3 deficient. Omega-3s in the diet can protect against cardiovascular heart disease, positively alter blood lipids, increase cardiac properties and vascular function and decrease inflammation.[3] The main chemicals in omega-3s that are thought to enhance health are eicosapentaenoic (EPA) and docosahexaenoic (DHA) acids. A number of plants and vegetables contain EPA and DHA, such as Chinese broccoli, flaxseed and spinach, but the highest amounts are contained in oily fish such as tuna, salmon and mackerel.

Protein

The third dangerous aspect of the modern diet is that we tend to eat too much of the wrong kinds of protein, namely red meat. For years, the food industry has convinced people that we must consume their products to get all the protein we need to be healthy. Protein, as the advertisements correctly point out, is an essential nutrient, but this emphasis on protein has created the idea that the only source of protein is from animal products. In Western societies, meals are primarily focused around meat. Our obsession with getting enough protein and eating animal products at almost every meal has created a situation of protein overload.[4] The notion that the only source of protein is meat and dairy is not true. In fact, all plant foods contain protein and it is possible to get all the protein you need from a strict vegetarian diet.[5] Consider the paradox whereby a cow grows quickly from a 20kg calf to a 360kg steer simply from the grass it eats.[6] It doesn't eat chicken or steak to get its protein. Even bigger is the African elephant, also a vegetarian. We do not need to eat meat or dairy products every day to get our protein, and the great majority of people who eat a lot of meat consume far too much protein.

Eating high levels of animal protein can cause health problems.[7] If we eat too much meat instead of vegetables, we are depriving ourselves of vital plant nutrients. Studies have shown that people who eat meat have twice the chance of dying from heart disease, 60% more chance of dying from cancer and 30% more chance of dying from other lifestyle diseases. There is now a plethora of research evidence supporting the health benefits of an unprocessed, plant-based diet. For example, it is now possible to create images of damaged heart arteries and then show that a plant-based diet reverses artherosclerosis. Ingesting meat proteins increases blood cholesterol levels in humans to a greater extent than consuming saturated fat. When diets of different countries are compared, results have shown that people consuming traditional plant-based diets experience significantly lower incidences of heart disease. In Westernised countries, people who consume more plant-based foods also have reduced incidence of heart disease. Vegetables such as asparagus, cauliflower, spinach, mung beans and broccoli have high levels of protein.[8] Nuts are also a great source of both protein and healthy fats. Almond, hazelnut, brazil nuts and cashews are all excellent sources of nutrition and are great to snack on when you feel hungry between meals. All nuts should be raw and free from any additive, such as salt.

Fibre

The fourth dangerous aspect of the modern diet is that we tend to eat too little fibre. Fibre is that portion of food that cannot be digested by enzymes in the human digestive tract and so does not provide any nutrients, but it plays a key role in regulating bowel activity. Nutritionists recommend that we eat at least 30 grams of fibre daily; unfortunately, most people in Western cultures only consume about half this amount. Fibre was first found to be important when physicians working in Africa noticed that those individuals who remained on traditional diets enjoyed very good health, but when they began eating refined grains and sugars, their health deteriorated. This discovery became known as the fibre hypothesis.

Studies have shown that those people who consume the most fibre have the lowest incidence of colorectal cancer. It has been estimated that if Americans increased their fibre intake by 13 grams a day from food sources – not as a supplement – about a third of all colorectal cancer in the USA could be avoided. However, it is not clear if this colorectal cancer prevention is solely due to high-fibre foods, because people eating this type of food typically eat less meat. Therefore, does eating meat increase risk of cancer or does consuming unprocessed food such as fruits and vegetables protect against cancer? A study in South Africa suggests that the much higher colon cancer rates among white compared to black South Africans may be because of the amount of animal protein and fat they eat rather than a deficiency in fibre intake. What is clear, however, is that diets naturally high in fibre and low in animal foods can prevent colon cancer.

The effects of dieting on belly fat and skeletal muscle

Severe dieting, such as cutting down the amount of food you eat by half, has been shown to result in weight loss in the short term, but most of this loss is in the form of body water and muscle protein. Some fat is typically lost but keeping this fat off is harder than losing it in the first place. Of those who lose body fat, over 90% will put the fat back on within 5 years.[9] There are also a number of unhealthy consequences that accompany severe dieting. The major problem is that cutting your daily calories in half for weeks or months will result in significant decreases in muscle mass. Skeletal muscle is very important for health and is one of the major tissues involved in fat burning; as mentioned, 1kg of muscle mass has the potential to burn up to an extra 3kg of fat per year. Other negative consequences that accompany severe dieting can include a reduced intake of essential minerals, vitamins and proteins, though these malnutrition aspects depend on the nature of the diet. Low-fat diets may also deprive individuals of healthy fats, such as the polyunsaturated or monounsaturated fats found in fish, olives, avocado and coconuts.

The 5 major problems with severe dieting are:

- a loss of muscle mass;
- reduced vitamins and minerals;
- a decrease in body water rather than body fat;
- reduced energy and increased fatigue; and
- constant hunger.

When it comes to belly fat and dieting, studies have shown that belly fat is easier to lose than subcutaneous fat. However, if you only cut the amount of calories you consume and don't exercise, you will lose some belly fat in the first 2–3 weeks but after that your belly fat loss will plateau.[10] The diets used in these studies have typically been starvation diets. Thus, the majority of diets, irrespective of their nature, are not sustainable in the long term, either because they are nutritionally poor or because they are tedious, difficult to carry out and expensive. What is needed instead is an eating plan that does not involve counting calories or starving yourself. Eating plans should be healthy but at the same time be fun and sustainable. A balanced eating plan should contain little junk food and processed food, small amounts of red meat, good fats and carbohydrates, and lots of plant protein. The eating plan we recommend is the Mediterranean eating plan.

The Mediterranean eating plan to help reduce belly fat

The Mediterranean eating plan is closely tied to areas of olive cultivation and involves eating lots of fruit and vegetables, beans, bread, nuts, whole-grain cereals, fish and seeds. White meat is eaten occasionally and red meat sparingly. Good fats, coconut, olive oil and omega-3s (fish oil) are consumed instead of saturated animal fat. Processed food is rarely eaten. A moderate amount of wine is consumed, usually with meals. A moderate amount of dark chocolate, a good source of antioxidants, is allowed, whereas junk and fried food is eliminated.

The cardioprotective effects of omega-3 fatty acids, polyphenols, oleic acid, natural antioxidants and folic acid, all contained in the Mediterranean eating plan, have been demonstrated.[11] Consumption of foods rich in arginine, an amino acid that is contained in nuts and fish, has been associated with decreased inflammation. High-fibre diets have also been associated with lowered inflammation levels. Inflammation is part of the body's immune response to something that enters or irritates our bodies. Inflammation often occurs when we pick up a bacterium or virus or when a joint gets injured after an accident or sporting injury. Inflammation can also occur by becoming overweight as a result of a lifestyle that involves little exercise and a diet consisting of lots of processed food.

Inflammation is detrimental to our health; it has been found that people with coronary artery disease typically have high levels of inflammation. The high medium-chain fatty acid content in olive oil has been shown to improve blood-fat profiles and reduce cardiovascular risk by reducing the amount of low-density lipoprotein cholesterol and enhancing the amount of high-density lipoprotein cholesterol found in the blood. Medium-chain fatty acid intake has also been shown to lower concentrations of insulin and glucose. Importantly, the Mediterranean eating plan works to improve health even if you don't happen to live in the Mediterranean area.[12]

How the Mediterranean eating plan works is unclear, but the fruit, vegetables and nuts in the program contain lots of phytonutrients that have high antioxidant and folic acid levels. There are also significant health benefits from consuming healthy fats, such as monounsaturated olive oil and the polyunsaturated omega-3s contained in fish oils.

How to calculate your Mediterranean eating score

Some people will have a number of Mediterranean foods already in their current diet, so it is useful to assess how much Mediterranean food you are eating. This can be done by calculating your Mediterranean eating score by answering the questions in the table on page 128.

To use the table, write a score in the right-hand column that reflects your typical diet. For the beneficial components, if you eat more than the average per day, your score is 1. For example, consuming more than 500 grams of vegetables per day would give you a score of 1. If you eat less than 500 grams of vegetables then your score would be 0. For the detrimental components, if you eat less than the average, your score would be 1. For example, 90 grams or less of meat per day would give you a score of 1. If you eat more than 90 grams of meat then your score would be 0.

Studies have shown that people experience significant health benefits after improving their score from 2 to 4, so health can be enhanced without having to achieve a perfect Mediterranean eating plan score of 8.

Diet component			
Beneficial components	**Average (per day)**	**The Mediterranean eating plan recommends**	**Score**
Vegetables	500g	Five average-sized servings	
Legumes	7g	One cup	
Fruits and nuts	360g	Four pieces of fruit and a handful of nuts	
Cereals	140g	One bowl of cereal	
Monounsaturated: saturated fat ratio	1:7		
Detrimental components	**Average (per day)**	**Guidelines**	**Score**
Meat and poultry	90g	Less than 1 chicken breast	
Dairy products	190g	Less than a glass of milk and 1 yoghurt	
Alcohol consumption *425ml in a schooner and 570ml in a pint	5–25g	Less than 2 schooners of beer*	

Adapted from Components of the MDS *(Trichopoulou, Costacou, Bamia & Trichopoulos, 2003).*[13]

Interpreting your score:

0–2 points: low levels of Mediterranean eating

3–4 points: moderately low levels of Mediterranean eating

5–6 points: moderately high levels of Mediterranean eating

7–8 points: high levels of Mediterranean eating

Mediterranean food

When cooking the Mediterranean way, grilling and boiling are the preferred methods.

Beans, peas and pastas
Beans contain lots of fibre, protein, healthy carbohydrates and iron. Most beans are also good sources of magnesium, which is important for heart health, and calcium, which is important for bone health. Healthy beans and peas include black-eyed peas, chick peas, green peas, lentils, snow peas and black, kidney, lima, pinto and navy beans.

Beans contain almost no fat and are low in calories. Sometimes called legumes, beans are one of the best plant sources of protein, fibre and iron. Because beans contain high levels of protein, a single serving can suppress your appetite for hours. Beans can also contribute to your daily fibre requirements. For example, there are approximately 8 grams of fibre in half a cup of cooked lentils, which amounts to about 25% of daily fibre needs. Unfortunately, most canned beans contain high levels of salt in the form of sodium. Check the nutrition label to make sure you only buy unsalted beans. Alternatively, buy dried beans and soak them according to packet instructions before cooking them.

Most pastas and noodles are full of simple carbohydrates and have little nutritional value. Processed pasta and noodles are also treated with a chlorine dioxide bleaching process, which destroys most nutrients. Over-processed noodles and pasta should be replaced with pasta and noodles like wholemeal pasta, spelt pasta, rice pasta, kamut pasta, quinoa pasta, ramen noodles, soba noodles and udon noodles.

Beverages

One glass for women and 2 for men of alcohol per day is permitted on the Mediterranean eating plan. All alcohol appears to have health benefits if taken in moderation.[14] Avoid sugary soft drinks and fruit juices as they contain refined sources of sugars, especially fructose. Replace soft drinks with water, green tea or coffee, which all have proven health benefits.

Chocolate

Dark chocolate and cocoa powder contains numerous antioxidants and high amounts of iron. One cup of cocoa powder provides about two-thirds of daily iron requirements. In contrast, a typical chocolate bar contains about 6% cocoa, so it is important to buy quality dark chocolate that consists of at least 70% cocoa if you need to satisfy a chocolate craving.

Dairy products

Low to moderate amounts of dairy foods, such as cheese, milk and yoghurt, are allowed on the Mediterranean eating plan. Low-fat or fat-free dairy foods should be used instead of full-fat versions.

Fats

The main fat used in the Mediterranean eating plan is olive oil, which has been shown to lower LDL (bad) cholesterol and increase HDL (good) cholesterol. Make sure to buy virgin or extra-virgin olive oil. Olive oil undergoes minimal processing so it retains its healthy plant antioxidants. In contrast, most other polyunsaturated oils, such as canola, safflower and corn oil, are heated and treated with solvents to improve their shelf life and appearance, which decreases their healthy plant compounds.

Fruits

Fruits are healthy and taste delicious. They contain lots of vitamins A and C and other health-supporting nutrients. People who consume 4–5 portions of fruit each day have low levels of heart disease, stroke and hypertension. Although the vitamins in fruit promote health, taking these exact vitamins in the form of supplements does not appear to enhance health as much. Fruit also contains fibre, minerals and antioxidants that, together with vitamins, work synergistically to protect against lifestyle diseases. All fruits are healthy but the following are nutrient-dense and appear to have the most disease-fighting potential: apples, bananas, blueberries, grapes, kiwis, oranges, papayas and strawberries. Other healthy fruits typically consumed on the Mediterranean eating plan are: cherries, dates, peaches, grapefruit and melon; most of these fruits contain high levels of vitamin C.

The majority of fruits have similar amounts of glucose and fructose. Apples and pears, however, contain more fructose than glucose. Fructose needs glucose to help it get out of the small intestine, therefore those people who eat a lot of apples and pears end up with fructose remaining in their small intestine. For some this situation causes colonisation of bacteria that cause problems such as abdominal pain and discomfort – these people are fructose-intolerant. To test if you are fructose-intolerant, stop eating apples and pears and drinking fruit juice or soft drink for 2 weeks and see if the discomfort goes away. If it does, then you are likely to be fructose-intolerant.

You should try to eat fresh fruits as much as possible. Unfortunately, the nutritional value of fruit can decrease rapidly if they are left for days in your house or do not arrive fresh to the supermarket. Chemicals such as pesticides are also used in fruit and vegetable farming to increase production, although the levels of these chemicals that are allowed in foods in most developed countries are considered safe. Pesticides are still toxic chemicals that kill agricultural pests, however, and they can cause health problems for humans if consumed in large amounts. If you want to avoid pesticides, buy organic food which is grown without the use of chemicals and pesticides.

Nuts and seeds

Nuts and seeds are another important part of the Mediterranean eating plan. About 80% of the calories in nuts come from fat, although the majority of fat in nuts is unsaturated. Nuts contain high calories, so try not to eat more than a handful per day. Healthy nuts include raw almonds, brazil nuts, cashews, pine nuts, hazelnuts, peanuts, pistachios and macadamias. Pumpkin, sesame, sunflower and flax seeds are also full of iron and other phyonutrients. All nuts and seeds should be unsalted and eaten raw.

Poultry and red meat

Neither poultry nor red meat should be consumed in high amounts when on the Mediterranean eating plan. Ideally, limit red meat to 1 or 2 meals per month. Although poultry appears to be healthier than red meat, it depends whether you are getting your chicken from a free range or a battery farm. Chickens reared on battery farms are abused animals, as they are typically packed by the thousands into massive, crowded sheds. They are fed large amounts of antibiotics and drugs to keep them alive, and these antibiotics make chickens grow large at an extremely fast rate. You only have to go to the supermarket and compare the size of a free-range chicken to a battery farm chicken to realise that something is wrong. A free-range chicken is always much smaller because it is not receiving antibiotics or being fed nutrients that increase its growth; if you want to eat chicken, make sure it is free-range. Chicken is a good source of protein, but when we eat beans, legumes, seeds and grains we can get protein, vitamins and iron in a much healthier form.

Seafood

When on the Mediterranean eating plan you should consume 2 servings of fish or shellfish per week, in place of red meat and poultry. Seafood typically consumed on the Mediterranean eating plan include: flounder, lobster, mackerel, mussels, oysters, prawn, salmon, squid and tuna.

Seasoning and spreads

In the Mediterranean eating plan, spices replace salt for seasoning. Spices typically consumed on the Mediterranean eating plan are: chilli, cinnamon, cloves, garlic, ginger, paprika, parsley, sage, saffron and turmeric. Two herbs that can be used to replace salt are garlic powder and freshly ground black pepper (not pre-ground pepper). Other options include onion powder (not onion salt). Butter and margarine are not used on the Mediterranean eating plan. You can replace them with coconut butter or nut butter.

Vegetables

Vegetables are a good source of protein, fibre, vitamin C, beta carotene, calcium and folate. Vegetables contain small amounts of calories but have high levels of nutrition. All vegetables are cholesterol free and nearly all contain no saturated fat; those that do usually have it in small amounts of healthy unsaturated fat. The energy in vegetables comes from a sugar called complex carbohydrate. Complex carbohydrate takes much more time to digest than simple carbohydrate, and consequently results in much lower levels of sugar (glucose) and insulin in the blood. However, some vegetables have a high glycemic index, which means that, when eaten, they result in high levels of sugar and insulin in the blood. High-glycemic vegetables include beetroot and corn.

When on the Mediterranean eating plan, around 5–7 servings of vegetables should be eaten every day. If you reduce your consumption of red meat then you should eat vegetables that are high in iron and vitamin C to prevent low iron levels, a condition known as anaemia. Vegetables containing high levels of iron are cooked Swiss chard, cooked turnip greens, raw kale and raw beetroot greens, whereas those with high vitamin C are broccoli, red and green chillis, capsicum, fresh thyme and parsley, and dark leafy vegetables such as kale and cress. Other healthy vegetables typically consumed on the Mediterranean eating plan are artichokes, celery, eggplant, lettuce, onions, peas, peppers, mushrooms, sweet potatoes and tomatoes. You should try to eat fresh vegetables whenever possible. Similar to fruit, the nutritional value of vegetables is reduced when they age on the shelf. The good news is that frozen vegetables and canned fruit contain about the same amount of healthy nutrients as when they are fresh.

Whole grains

The grains that you eat should be whole grains that contain no saturated or trans fats. Whole grains typically consumed on the Mediterranean eating plan are oats, barley, buckwheat, bulgur wheat, couscous, millet and rice. All these grains contain high levels of iron.

It is best not to eat processed cereals as they are nutritionally poor. If you have to eat a commercial breakfast cereal then check its nutritional information panel first, as they typically contain high levels of sugar in the form of fructose.

Sample recipes for a Mediterranean breakfast, dinner and lunch

There are hundreds of Mediterranean recipes and cooking tips available on recipe websites like www.taste.com.au, www.lifestylefood.com.au and www.eatingwell.com, and an extensive number of healthy Mediterranean recipes are also to be found in books like *Ultrametabolism* by Dr Mark Hyman and *Belly Fat Weight Loss* by Claire Wheeler and Diane A. Welland. Below you'll find a sample menu of recipes suitable for breakfast, lunch and dinner. Each recipe serves 1 person, unless otherwise stated.

Breakfast

Scrambled eggs and toast

A good Mediterranean breakfast is scrambled eggs on whole-grain toast. Butter or margarine should not be used on the toast. Going without butter may be difficult, but coconut or nut butter can be used as a healthy substitute. This meal can be followed by whole fruit such as an orange or a slice of melon. Drink unsweetened Sencha green tea, black tea, coffee or water; do not drink fruit juice as it contains high concentrations of fructose.

You will need:

    2 eggs

    1 tablespoon low-fat or skim milk

    1 teaspoon freshly ground black pepper, or spice of your choice

Method

1. Beat the eggs with the milk and freshly ground black pepper
2. Pour mixture into a heated non-stick fry pan. As the egg at the edge of the pan sets, pull it back to the centre and allow the uncooked egg to move to the edge of the pan so the egg scrambles.
3. Serve scrambled eggs on whole-grain toast.

Fruit, nuts, and yoghurt

This breakfast is quick to prepare and can contain a range of fruit and nuts. The yoghurt should be non-fat or low-fat Greek.

You will need:

½–1 cup fruit of your choice, such as banana, melon, berries, mango, apple or pear

½ cup low-fat, low-sugar yoghurt

½ cup chopped raw, unsalted nuts of your choice, such as almonds, cashews or hazelnuts

Method

1. Chop larger fruit into smaller pieces but keep fruit whole whenever possible. Place fruit in a cereal bowl.
2. Cover fruit with yoghurt. Sprinkle chopped raw nuts over the yoghurt.

Cereal and fruit (serves 2)

As most commercial cereals contain high levels of sugar, it is best if you make your own. Adding blueberries, chopped bananas and peaches to a healthy home-made cereal creates a great breakfast. Use low-fat milk, but

if you don't like cow's milk, try a non-dairy milk such as coconut, rice or soy. If you don't want to consume any form of milk, then add fresh fruit and yogurt to the cereal as per the recipe on page 138.

You will need:

>   2 tablespoons sunflower seeds
>
>   4 tablespoons sliced almonds
>
>   2 tablespoons chopped nuts of your choice, such as almonds, cashews, or hazelnuts
>
>   1½ cups rolled oats
>
>   2 tablespoons sultanas or your preferred dried fruit
>
>   1 teaspoon cinnamon

Method

1. Place sunflower seeds, sliced almonds and chopped to rolled oats in a bowl and mix well.
2. To sweeten, add the sultanas and cinnamon.
3. Serve with low-fat milk or yoghurt and top with the fruit of your choice.

Lunch

Curried vegetables

Any vegetable can be used in this recipe, however harder vegetables such as carrots and potatoes should be precooked.

You will need:

- 1 tablespoon olive oil
- 1 cup chopped mixed vegetables, such as asparagus, onion, potato, carrot, broccoli, peas or capsicum
- 2 eggs
- 1 teaspoon curry powder

Method

1. Place olive oil in a frying pan over medium heat. Add vegetables and stir-fry for 3 minutes.
2. Beat the eggs in a bowl and add curry powder.
3. Add eggs to the vegetables and cook for 3 minutes, stirring occasionally until the eggs are cooked.

Spicy burrito (serves 4)

Beans are extremely healthy (if you buy the canned, no-salt variety) and quick to prepare. Multiple toppings can be used to generate many different flavours and this burrito can be spiced up by adding chilli powder and cayenne pepper.

You will need:

- 1 tablespoon of olive oil
- 1 onion, chopped
- 1 red capsicum, chopped

400g tin no-salt kidney or mixed beans

1 clove garlic, crushed

¼ teaspoon chilli powder

¼ teaspoon cayenne pepper

½ cabbage, shredded

1 tomato, diced, seeds removed

½ red onion, diced

1 teaspoon chopped coriander

1 teaspoon lime juice

freshly ground black pepper, to taste

1 tablespoon low-fat sour cream

4 tortillas

Method

1. Put olive oil in a frying pan and place over medium heat.

2. Sauté onion and capsicum for 5 minutes, turning occasionally, until soft and onion is transparent.

3. Add beans, garlic, chilli powder and cayenne pepper and sauté for another 10 minutes.

4. Meanwhile, place cabbage, tomato, red onion coriander, lime juice, black pepper and sour cream in a bowl and mix thoroughly. Heat tortillas in the oven.

5. Divide the bean mixture between the tortillas and top with the cabbage salsa, then roll each tortilla to create the burritos.

Dinner

Roasted salmon with asparagus

This meal combines healthy salmon with asparagus.
You will need:

    2 tablespoons macadamia nuts, crushed

    2 tablespoons coriander, chopped

    1 tablespoon coconut butter

    1 teaspoon lemon zest

    170 gram piece of fresh salmon

    freshly ground black pepper, to taste

    6 asparagus spears

    1 tablespoon Parmesan shavings

    Lemon slices, to serve

Method

1. Pre-heat oven to 230°C.

2. Combine macadamia nuts and coriander in a bowl. Add the coconut butter and lemon zest to the macadamia and coriander and mix well.

3. Place salmon on a tray, skin-side down and season with freshly ground black pepper. Spread macadamia and coriander mix thickly over the salmon flesh. Place in the oven and roast for 12–16 minutes, until just cooked.

4. While your salmon is roasting, preheat the grill to medium. Place asparagus spears on a baking tray, drizzle with olive oil and place under the grill for 3–4 minutes.

5. Place asparagus spears on a plate and cover with parmesan shavings and freshly ground black pepper. Place the salmon fillet on top of the asparagus spears and garnish with lemon slices.

Lemon caper chicken

Serve this meal with sautéed whole greens of your choice.

You will need:

- 1 small chicken breast, trimmed of all fat
- freshly ground black pepper, to taste
- 1 tablespoon olive oil
- zest and juice of half a lemon
- ¼ cup chicken stock
- ½ cup couscous
- ¼ cup chopped fresh parsley leaves
- 1 clove garlic, crushed
- 65g cherry tomatoes, quartered
- 1 tablespoon drained capers
- 1 spring onion, sliced

Method

1. Place chicken breast, pepper, garlic and olive oil in a shallow dish and mix to combine.

2. Heat a medium saucepan over medium-high heat and then add the chicken mixture. Cook for 2-3 minutes while tossing the mixture until almost cooked. Transfer to a plate and keep warm by covering the plate with foil.

3. Increase heat to high and add lemon juice and stock. Cook until the liquid comes to a boil and then remove saucepan and add couscous. Make sure none of the mixture sticks to the bottom of the pan. Cover and let stand for 2–3 minutes.
4. Now add the chicken, tomatoes, parsley, green onion, capers and lemon zest. Combine and serve.

How to switch to the Mediterranean eating plan

Beginning the Mediterranean eating plan is simple and will soon become habit if you follow it for 6 weeks. First, stop consuming all junk and fried foods and soft drinks and only consume fruit juice in moderation. Replace red meat with white meat, such as free-range chicken and fish, and with tofu. Drink only filtered water and green tea. Cut down saturated fat so it forms less than 8% of your total calories, although you can use coconut oil occasionally as it is a healthy form of saturated fat. Use the good fats, such as olive oil and those containing omega-3s more frequently – they should be about 20–30% of your daily calories. Use a fish oil supplement – one that gives you about 1.8 grams per day is best – if you are not eating lots of fish or seafood or are concerned about toxins. Replace sweets and sugary foods with fruit and low-fat, low-sugar yogurt. For example, an orange contains only 77 calories of energy but provides over 4 grams of fibre and lots of other nutrients, such as vitamin C. In contrast, a typical chocolate bar contains no fibre or helpful nutrients but contains about 238 calories – over 3 times more energy than the orange. Drink wine in moderation, consuming only 1 glass per day for women and 2 glasses per day for men. Replace milk chocolate with an extra-fine dark chocolate that has at least 70% cocoa, and eat it sparingly. After 6 weeks you should have more energy and vitality, and for most people there will be no need to count calories.

Although changing eating habits can be challenging, following the 4 steps below should increase your chance of converting to a healthy Mediterranean eating plan. And if all this sounds complicated, consult a dietician.

- Identify Mediterranean foods. Read the previous section and seek out more detailed information from the resources mentioned.

- The majority of your eating plan should involve consuming healthy fruits, vegetables, whole grains, nuts and beans. Processed foods such as fried chips and meat, soft drinks, margarine, cakes and biscuits should be eliminated.

- Replace red meat mostly with fish and some free-range chicken and turkey. Limit your consumption of red meat to 2 portions per month.

- Use olive oil as your major fat. This is a healthy fat and should be used liberally.

How to keep the fat off

Let's say you lose body fat by adopting the Mediterranean eating plan and the interval sprinting program described in Chapter 3. How do you then keep it off? Unfortunately, keeping fat off is more difficult than losing it in the first place. As mentioned, over 90% of people who lose body fat by dieting will put it back on again after 5 years.[15] The difficulty in maintaining body fat loss is that continuing with dieting and exercise is extremely challenging for most people. A tiny percentage of people, however, don't regain the fat they've lost. Not much was known about keeping fat off until the National Weight Control Registry (NWCR) was established in the US in the late 1990s. The NWCR is a database of over 5000 people who have lost a minimum of 13.6kg of weight and have kept it off for at least 12 months. Average weight loss in the NWCR is 30kg, and the average period of weight loss is greater than 5 years.[16] This group of people volunteered to be monitored to help show what really is important for long-term weight control.

The NWCR study discovered that those people who were successful in keeping body fat off shared 6 healthy habits:

- They had an healthy eating plan and exercised regularly;
- They ate breakfast every day;
- They stayed clear of fast food;
- They reduced their energy intake by eating a low-saturated-fat diet;
- They followed a consistent eating plan; and
- They reduced their TV watching hours.

As we can see, people who are successful in keeping fat off eat healthily, exercise regularly and always eat breakfast. An interesting characteristic of the NWCR people was that they averaged less than 1 fast food meal per week, including restaurant meals; even in restaurants that provide healthier food, there are still concerns about salt levels and overheating and repeated use of cooking oils. As would be expected, most people in the NWCR had a diet that was low-calorie with low-saturated-fat content. Reducing energy intake, however, does not mean eating less food. Staying away from energy-rich foods allows you to enjoy more of the delicious, healthy dishes contained in a Mediterranean eating plan.

Those who followed a consistent, structured eating plan maintained more weight loss. This is because flexible, spontaneous eating plans offer more opportunities to eat highly processed, unhealthy foods. The

NWCR study and a number of others have shown that those who watch a lot of TV are typically overweight. Therefore, substituting some TV time with physical activity would be helpful for maintaining fat loss.

Nutrients that enhance or impede fat burning

Our studies have shown that nutritional patterns make a difference to how successful losing belly fat through interval sprinting is: what you consume when attempting to lose fat by exercising may decrease or enhance fat burning. Some individuals may have an eating plan that includes lots of healthy, unprocessed foods, such as fruit, vegetables and fish, which enhance fat burning, while others may consume processed foods, such as soft drinks and sweets, that contain high levels of fructose or other refined products, which suppress fat burning.

Nutrients that enhance fat burning typically affect the fat-burning hormones or their cell receptors. For example, green tea ingestion results in enhanced fat burning by blocking enzymes that degrade norepinephrine. Norepinephrine and epinephrine are the major fat-burning hormones and are responsible for releasing fat from fat cells and inducing fat burning in tissues such as the liver and skeletal muscle. A catechin present in green tea called epigallocatechin gallate (EGCG) appears to be responsible for this effect. An *American*

Journal of Clinical Nutrition article showed that drinking 4 cups of green tea a day resulted in a loss of more than 6 pounds (2.7kg) in 8 weeks. However, other clinical trials have not shown a fat-loss effect after green tea consumption. Caffeine also induces fat burning, but does so by elevating sympathetic nervous activity, which elevates levels of epinephrine in the blood, and by blocking the adenosine receptors on fat cells that suppress fat release. Research has shown that drinking 500ml of cold water can increase metabolic rate by a third, mainly due to an increase in fat-releasing hormones such as norepinephrine. Drinking 2 cups of warm rather than cold water resulted in a much smaller increase in metabolic rate.

Consuming omega-3 fatty acids may also contribute to fat loss by triggering fat-burning enzymes inside cells. Omega-3s also appear to improve leptin signalling in the brain, which reduces appetite. Cold-water fish such as tuna and salmon are good sources of omega-3, as are nuts, seeds and flaxseed, which contain fats that are changed to omega-3s when ingested.

Capsaicin, the compound that makes chillis hot, has also been shown to enhance fat burning. Most of the research examining the fat-burning effect of chillis has administered the capsaicin in capsule form, which has been found to be more effective than when it's contained in food. The mechanisms underlying the capsaicin effect are unclear but are likely to include an increase in energy expenditure, impeded fat-cell growth and a reduction in appetite. Capsaicin can be obtained naturally by consuming raw, cooked, dried or powdered chillis and capsicums. Cayenne pepper or hot sauce can also be added to home-made soups and meals.

We think other nutrients and minerals may enhance or impede fat burning indirectly. For example, having low levels of iron is associated with a slower metabolism, resulting in less fat burning. So correcting low iron levels – anaemia – can improve the body's ability to burn fat; 1 cup of lentils provides about 35% of daily iron needs.

The thyroid gland affects every cell in the body and has a significant impact on metabolism and fat loss or gain, immunity, hormones, heart rate and blood pressure. Thyroid dysfunction often has a genetic influence; it isn't unusual for grandparents, parents and children to all possess thyroid dysfunction. However, nutrients in food can also increase or decrease thyroid function. For example, iodised salt contains iodine, which is essential for thyroid function. Avoiding table salt and consuming little iodine is likely to result in a depressed thyroid in most people. Processed foods typically contain lots of salt but not the iodised kind. Meat and chicken typically contain antibiotics and growth stimulants that have been shown to reduce thyroid function. Surprisingly, some vegetables impede iodine absorption, resulting in reduced thyroid function. Such vegetables usually contain a chemical called goitrogen however cooking typically negates this goitrogen effect. Thyroid-reducing vegetables include green leafy vegetables such as raw cabbage, broccoli and spinach. Soy also contains goitrogens, and studies have shown that although it is thought of as a healthy food, soy is detrimental for thyroid function; it follows that cooking oils and margarine that contain soybean should be avoided. Replace oils containing soybean with coconut oil and extra-virgin olive oil. Kelp contains high levels of iodine and, in contrast to soy, has been shown to improve thyroid function.

The status of your thyroid needs to be medically evaluated, which typically involves an assessment of the thyroid hormones in your blood by a doctor knowledgeable in endocrinology. Hypothyroidism refers to a thyroid gland that is underperforming, whereas hyperthyroidism reflects an overactive thyroid.

Most processed foods suppress fat burning. These include anything that has been deep-fried, soft drinks, milk chocolate, margarine, cakes and biscuits, pies, donuts, take-away burgers, hot dogs, sausages and so forth. The mechanism underlying the fat-burning suppression of these foods is most likely that processed foods take fewer calories to digest than unprocessed food. One study indicated that people burned fewer calories after eating a processed meal rather than a meal comprised of whole foods. Researchers first gave volunteers a cheddar cheese sandwich on whole-grain bread, then, on a second day, a processed cheese sandwich on white bread. Both sandwiches had the same amount of calories. The metabolic rate of the subjects was measured and revealed that 137 calories were burned after eating the sandwich made with cheddar cheese, compared to 73 calories after eating the processed cheese sandwich. In this case, unprocessed food resulted in the burning of 43% more calories.

The replacement of processed foods with whole foods results in burning more calories due to what is called the thermic effect of eating whole foods. The cheese sandwiches made with whole-grain bread contained high levels of fibre, too, which lowers the surge in blood insulin levels that occurs with eating; high levels of insulin after a meal decrease fat burning. Do what you can to avoid these foods and replace them with healthy eating, such as the Mediterranean eating plan.

Nutrients that reduce fat absorption

A number of nutrients have an effect on the amount of fat we absorb from what we eat. For example, ingestion of oolong tea – a form of green tea – with a high-fat meal significantly lowered fat absorption.[17] One study showed that the amount of total lipids and cholesterol remaining in the faecal mass of subjects increased by 52% after drinking 750ml of oolong tea each meal per day. The healthy components of green tea are called catechins, which are powerful antioxidants. Green tea contains many catechins, although epigallocatechin gallate (EGCG) seems to be responsible for the greatest lipid absorption effect. EGCG suppresses the uptake of lipids in the small intestine and is also effective at lowering the absorption of cholesterol.

It has also been found that green tea lowers the absorption of organic pollutants, which humans can easily absorb. This leads to high levels of tissue toxicity and the prevention of fat loss. For example, eating trans fats and oxidised and polyunsaturated vegetable oils results in increased accumulation of free radicals in our bodies. Free radicals are atoms with an odd number of electrons and are typically created when oxygen interacts with other molecules. Free radicals cause damage by reacting with the DNA inside our cells, resulting in cell death and disease. Antioxidants can prevent the negative effects of free radicals by terminating their ability to damage cells. To help the body produce enough antioxidants, a diet containing vitamins such as beta-carotene, vitamin C and vitamin E is necessary.

Eating fruit and plants containing insect pesticides can also result in a build-up of toxins in adipose cells. The accumulated toxins inside the adipose cell can be released when stimulated, which has been shown to slow fat loss and therefore may make people fat. Green tea prevents absorption of organic pollutants, so people who regularly drink green tea may experience more fat loss by reducing fat absorption in the meals they eat and by decreasing the toxicity effect of organic pollutants.

Fat and sugar in the blood after eating a meal

Eating 3 meals per day containing 20–40 grams of saturated fat or 50 grams of fructose typically causes elevated triglyceride blood levels lasting up to 18 hours. This phenomenon is called postprandial lipemia and is a major risk factor for atherosclerosis and cardiovascular disease, because higher levels of fat in the blood increase inflammation and disrupt the lining of the arteries.

Postprandial lipemia levels vary, but they are decreased or increased by food intake, fat type, dietary intake of protein, nutrients and exercise. For example, consuming 30 grams or more of saturated fat typically results in postprandial lipemia, whereas eating monounsaturated and polyunsaturated fats does not. Consuming protein, fibre and green tea with saturated fat results in lowered postprandial lipemia, whereas drinking alcohol and smoking enhances it.[18]

One session of aerobic exercise lasting 45 minutes resulted in significantly lower postprandial lipemia. People regularly performing aerobic exercise every week also exhibit lower postprandial lipemia. Recently, our studies have shown that 20 minutes of interval sprinting at night also reduced fat in the blood of women who ate a high-fat meal the next morning.[19]

Postprandial lipemic individuals can be inflamed for a significant proportion of the day, and this inflamed state is likely to impede fat loss. Inflammation raises insulin and cortisol levels; these are hormones that enhance fat storing. Therefore, eating meals high in saturated fat may increase belly fat stores to a greater extent than eating less saturated fat or consuming healthier fats. Those individuals who ingest high-saturated-fat meals but consume protein, fibre or green tea simultaneously may experience a suppressed postprandial lipemia and inflammatory response.

Eating lots of simple sugar can also cause postprandial elevations in glucose, which in turn can increase inflammation, endothelial dysfunction and hyperinsulinaemia. Eating healthy foods such as vegetables, fruits, seeds, grains and nuts results in a far lower rate of postprandial glucose elevation.[20] Drinking 1–2 glasses of alcohol before eating a high-sugar meal also results in significantly lower postprandial glucose levels, and drinking a moderate amount of alcohol decreases insulin resistance for 12–24 hours. Consuming olive oil and fish oil significantly lowers postprandial plasma glucose levels, and such reduction in postprandial glucose levels leads to decreased blood insulin levels. As previously discussed, insulin enhances fat storage, and high blood insulin levels are an impediment to fat loss. Therefore, as discussed with postprandial lipemia, ingestion of different types of nutrients with a meal that affect postprandial glucose and insulin could influence belly fat loss response.

What to eat before, during and after exercising

Digesting nutrients before, during and after exercising influences fat burning. Eating 30 grams of fructose or glucose 1 hour before a 60-minute aerobic exercise session significantly suppressed whole body fat burning by 32% (fructose) and 50% (glucose). Unfortunately, consuming a high-protein meal also results in a significant increase in blood insulin levels. It is important not to eat sugar or protein before or immediately after exercise, as these nutrients elevate blood insulin levels, which impair fat burning. Digesting low-glycemic meals before exercise also suppresses fat oxidation, but the effect is much greater after high-glycemic meals. Low-glycemic meals contain fewer simple sugars, such as glucose, whereas high-glycemic meals contain lots of glucose; consuming sugary drinks and protein snacks before or after exercise will tend to suppress fat burning and reduce long-term fat loss.

In contrast, other nutrients can enhance fat burning during and after exercise. For example, we have shown that ingestion of green tea before interval sprinting increased fat oxidation by over 20% during the hour after exercise.[21] Another study demonstrated that green tea ingestion before steady-state cycle aerobic exercise resulted in a 17% increase in fat oxidation during exercise.[22]

Time of day for optimal belly fat loss with interval sprinting exercise

The time of day you choose to exercise and whether or not you have eaten a meal before your session affects fat burning during exercise. Studies have shown exercising following an overnight fast results in significantly greater fat burning during exercise, compared to exercising soon after a meal.

One such study also investigated the effect of exercise on glucose intolerance and insulin resistance in the fasted and fed states.[23] It found that fasted training was more effective than fed training for improving glucose tolerance and insulin resistance: fasted compared to fed subjects displayed the greatest insulin sensitivity levels. The fasted subjects also significantly increased fat burning, which resulted in a much smaller weight increase in the fasted group. Thus, even though they consumed a high-caloric diet, fasted subjects gained much less weight after the 6-week program. This and other studies have shown that the body burns up much more fat during and after exercise if no food is eaten before exercise. This means the best time of day to exercise in order to lose belly fat is early in the morning, before breakfast.

Exercise and appetite

Overall, the evidence indicates that engaging in exercise does not automatically increase appetite; with most people who exercise, food intake remains unchanged, and in certain circumstances exercise may suppress appetite. It is possible that exercising may change the quality of nutrients eaten; for example, after hot, sweaty exercise there may be a switch away from high-fat foods to fruit and water. However, this has not been examined thoroughly and is an important future research area.

Hard exercise, such as running a marathon, has been shown to induce a moderate decrease in appetite, lasting up to several hours after the session, but moderate exercise does not seem to have any effect on appetite. When people change from a sedentary lifestyle to an active one, food intake is not increased accordingly, which seems to suggest there is no biological mechanism that matches energy output to energy intake; rather, social and psychological factors may determine how much and what we eat.

The mechanisms underlying the appetite-suppressant effect incurred by hard, vigorous exercise are unknown, but increased body temperature may inhibit food intake; people in cold climates normally eat more than those in temperate or warm regions. Recent research has also shown that a number of gut peptides change after exercise and may inhibit food intake by suppressing central nervous system appetite circuits.[24] Other studies have shown that satiety hormones released from the brain during hard exercise also suppress appetite, and that elevated blood lactate levels blunt appetite by affecting appetite centres in the brain.[25] In contrast, however, other studies have shown that cold-water workouts increase appetite – individuals who exercise in cool water eat more afterwards.[26] The effect of interval sprinting on appetite has not been examined and is an important area for future research, but we already know lactate levels are increased in the blood during interval sprinting.

Successful fat loss involves a lifestyle change, *not* short-term starvation. The components of healthy living – healthy eating, exercise, a reasonable amount of stress and quality sleep – all interact to influence our body composition and health. The Mediterranean eating plan is ideal for individuals living in the Western industrialised world, as it requires minimal preparation and does not involve counting calories. Combined with exercise and stress-management, it provides the basis for a healthy lifestyle.

*

This chapter has emphasised what we should be eating. The ideal way to eat for optimum health includes:

- avoiding processed foods with added sugar;
- consuming those saturated fats that are good for health (coconut, avocado), while eliminating those saturated fats that are bad for health;
- consuming those polyunsaturated and monounsaturated oils that are good for health (olive oil, fish oil), while elimintaing those polyunsaturated fats, such as vegetable oils, that are bad for health;
- eating plants full of fibre (apples, coconut, strawberries);
- reducing or eliminating animal protein, as too much is bad for health, and replacing it with beneficial plant proteins; and
- following the Mediterranean eating plan, as it is the only diet that that has documented beneficial clinical outcomes.

The right kind of exercise, combined with a healthy, nutritious eating program, is a step in the right direction to losing belly fat and keeping it off. But these are not the only factors that lead to fat gain. Our busy modern lives mean we are more stressed and sleeping less, both factors that encourage our bodies to put on dangerous belly fat. Chapter 5 looks at ways of managing your levels of stress and how to get enough sleep to gain the full benefit from your 20x3 belly-fat reduction program.

Chapter 5
Reducing daily stress and enhancing sleep quality

What is stress?

Stress is a process that happens when people respond to environmental and psychological stressors that generate challenge or danger. Stress stimulates the 'fight or flight' centres in the brain, which brings about the release of stress hormones such as catecholamines and cortisol. The catecholamines called epinephrine and norepinephrine increase our breathing rate to provide more oxygen to muscles, elevate heart rate and blood pressure and mobilise fat into the blood for extra energy. Muscles also can become tense, and a decrease in saliva flow and increase in sweat production can be experienced. Cortisol, another stress hormone, helps store fat and releases sugar into the blood.

The stress response is not always generated by the situation alone – the anticipation of a potential stressor can also have a significant impact on how stress affects an individual. A small amount of stress can add interest to daily life and can help us adapt to change, but too much stress has been shown to cause a range of health problems and an increase in belly fat.

Types of stressors include cataclysmic, personal and daily. A cataclysmic stressor occurs infrequently but is typically life-changing. For example, civil wars, tornadoes and tsunamis cause great disruption to people's lives and can typically bring about a significant stress response. Personal stressors are usually infrequent but can be equally stressful; the death of a loved one or undergoing a divorce has been shown to generate a significant stress response. Daily stressors involve the frustrations that many of us experience, such as commuting in busy traffic, working with people perceived to be incompetent, having too much work to complete in too little time and so forth. These stressors can occur frequently throughout the day and have the ability to constantly generate a stress response, which can lead to a number of health problems, such as increased incidence of heart attacks, gastrointestinal problems, hypertension, stroke, diabetes, cancer, tuberculosis, insomnia, pneumonia, influenza and headaches.

The effect of stress on belly fat

The major stress hormone that affects belly fat is cortisol; high levels of cortisol in the blood lead to increased deposits of belly fat. Enhanced blood cortisol levels make the liver release sugar into the blood, bringing about an increase in blood insulin levels. Constant high levels of cortisol and insulin in the blood encourage fat accumulation and an increase in belly fat, so individuals exposed to stressors may increase their belly fat stores due to their elevated cortisol and insulin levels.

There is a link between stress, cortisol and appetite, as studies have shown that injecting people with cortisol caused increased appetite and sugar ingestion. Young women who secreted more cortisol during stress also consumed more sugar and fat afterwards. Cortisol may influence appetite by binding to receptors in the hypothalamus, a part of the brain that controls appetite. This can cause people to consume more junk foods, which contain large amounts of fat and sugar. Cortisol also regulates other chemicals that control appetite. For example, stress hormones such as corticotropin-releasing hormone and neuropeptide Y have been shown to stimulate appetite. Exposure to stressors also elevates inflammation levels, which have been implicated in the development of obesity.

Measuring your daily stress

The amount of daily stress in your life can be assessed in the test below. If you score more than 20 points, you have high levels of stress and need to take action to reduce your daily stress levels. To assess your typical daily stress levels, answer the 6 questions using a score between 1 and 4 for each question, and then sum your total.

1 = Not at all   2 = Sometimes
3 = Fairly regularly   4 = All the time

1. I worry about personal problems in my life every day

2. My personal problems interfere with my job and relationships

3. I constantly feel that things in my life are out of control

4. I feel the stress in my life affects my health

5. I find the stress in my life disrupts my sleep

6. I often feel anxious and irritable during the day

TOTAL

Interpreting your score:
6-9 points: low levels of daily stress
10-12 points: moderately low levels of daily stress
13-18 points: moderately high levels of daily stress
19-24 points: high levels of daily stress

How to cope with stress

There are a number of ways to cope with stress, including taking direct action against and seeking information about the stressor, inhibiting stressful actions and employing general stress-management habits. For example, if a person's job is their main source of stress, then the best solution would be to find another job. Unfortunately, for most people this is not practical, so they have to find a way of coping with the stress generated by their jobs. If driving in morning traffic is stressful, then a way to cope might be to get information about traffic flow during different times of the day, to provide options for decreasing the stressful effects of traffic.

Another coping mechanism is to stop fighting the stressor and accept it – this is called inhibiting the stressor. It does not get rid of the stressors but saves the energy and effort required for coping with them. For example, rather than getting angry and upset every time you get involved in morning traffic, you could accept that city roads will always be busy and play music rather than get upset.

Finally, if a stressor cannot be removed or inhibited, then stress-management offers a number of strategies and techniques to reduce or stop the deleterious effects of exposure to daily stressors. Read on and learn how to use stress-management skills such as controlled breathing, muscle relaxation and imagery to avoid becoming agitated.

Stress-management

Stress-management typically involves managing stressors where possible, modifying appraisal of stressful situations, developing stress resistance resources, controlling stress reactions, controlled breathing, muscle relaxation and imagery. More information on these strategies can be found in *Minding the Body, Mending the Mind* by Joan Borysenko.[1] From a belly fat perspective, the most important strategies include the use of exercise and the development of controlled breathing, muscle relaxation, imagery and time-management skills to cope with stress.

Controlled breathing

Controlled breathing is a stress-management technique that concentrates on slowing and optimising your breathing. Rapid breathing quickly produces a number of negative physiological responses, such as an elevated heart rate and disrupted cardiac autonomic activity.

A warm, darkened, carpeted room is recommended when learning how to control your breathing and muscle tension. You should lie on your back with your arms by your side; you can lie on the floor or a firm bed. Make sure your clothing is not tight or uncomfortable. Finally, make sure you do not have any injuries that cause discomfort when lying in this position. Now follow the steps listed below.

1. Focus your thoughts on your breathing.

2. Slow your breathing and take deep, even breaths. Focus all your thoughts on the air as it enters your nasal passage and progresses deep into your lungs. If extraneous thoughts enter your mind, push them aside and refocus all your attention on your breathing.

3. Now concentrate on your breathing cue word: RELAX. As you say the word in your mind, breathe in on the *RE* and out on the *LAX*. One cycle should take about 5 seconds – 2.5 seconds breathing in, and 2.5 seconds breathing out – which equates to 12 breathing cycles per minute. Practise using this cue for 3 breathing cycles. Remember, slowly breathe in on the *RE* and slowly breathe out on the *LAX*.

4. If thoughts enter your mind or noises come to your attention, push them aside and refocus all your concentration on your breathing.

5. As you prastice the muscle relaxation technique in the next section, try to monitor and control your breathing throughout the session using your cue word, RELAX.

Muscle relaxation

Muscle relaxation is a technique that systematically releases all the tension in your skeletal muscles. As with the controlled breathing technique, you should lie on your back with arms by your side in a warm, darkened room. Try to wear comfortable, non-restrictive clothing. Follow the instructions below to learn how muscle relaxation is performed for the whole body.

1. Lie on your back on a carpeted floor or on a firm bed. Support your head with a small cushion. Allow your legs and arms to stretch out. If you suffer from lower-back problems, place a rolled-up blanket under the backs of your knees.

2. To begin, complete a body tension check by monitoring all your muscle groups for excessive muscle tension. Close your eyes and scan the muscles in your body from your head to your feet. Try to assess which of your muscles are tense. Don't forget about your breathing; it should be slow and even.

3. Now start muscle relaxation: tense your fist by curling your fingers as tight as you can for 15 seconds. Hold the tension and focus on it, then release by relaxing your hands and letting your fingers slowly uncurl. Notice the warm, tingling

feeling of relaxed muscles, compared to the earlier feeling of tension.

4. Next, focus on your biceps. Create tension in these muscles for 15 seconds by lifting both hands to the shoulders and tightening the biceps. Try to keep your hands relaxed. Now release the tension in your biceps by relaxing them and letting your arms slowly return to your side.

5. Now tense your neck muscles by contracting and pushing the back of your neck into the pillow for 15 seconds. Hold the tension, focus on it, then release it by relaxing your neck.

6. Tense your facial muscles by frowning and gritting your teeth for 15 seconds. Hold the tension, focus on it, then release it by relaxing.

7. Now contract you abdominal muscles by tensing and pulling your stomach towards your spine for 15 seconds. Hold the tension, focus on it, then release it by relaxing.

8. Next continue with your thighs and buttocks. Tense these muscles tightly for 15 seconds, then release the tension.

9. Don't forget your breathing. Focus on your breathing by using your cue word, RELAX.

Take a deep breath on the *RE*, hold your breath, then release it on the *LAX*.

10. Finish by tensing your lower legs. Keep your eyes closed and contract your feet and lower legs by pushing them into the carpet or bed. Hold the tension for 15 seconds, then relax. By now you should feel your body getting warm and heavy.

11. Once you have completed the exercise, remain lying down for a while. You may go to sleep, so if you have other things to do, set an alarm clock before you begin.

Imagery relaxation

Much stress is caused by thinking about negative situations, so for some people relaxing muscles may not be enough and they must also relax their minds by blocking stressful thoughts and trying to stop worrying. Relaxation imagery involves imagining a relaxing scene by using sight, sound, smell and touch, which distracts a stressed person from worrying.

Choose a relaxing image that you most associate with calmness, peace, tranquility, serenity and harmony. It may be a real-life scenario, such as walking through countryside, or a fantasy image, such as drifting along with the clouds in the sky. Try to involve all your senses in your image, so think about what you can see, hear, touch and smell. The 2 practice images described in the instructions below involve clouds and a warm house in winter. Try these images and then develop your own.

When practising relaxation imagery, a warm, darkened, carpeted room is recommended. You should lie on your back with your arms by your side. Make sure your clothing is not tight or uncomfortable. Also make sure you do not have any injuries that cause you discomfort when lying in this position.

Now create the flowing scene in your mind. You are on a warm, white beach. You are the only one on the beach and the water is calm and green, and the sky is a vivid blue. Focus on the sky. In your mind's eye, you see nothing but blue. Now focus on the green and turquoise colours of the sea. Focus on the smell of the ocean, let the fresh smell of the sea flood your mind. You can feel a gentle sea breeze blowing against your face. Next, focus on the sky, where you can see a small white cloud slowly descending to the beach. The cloud becomes larger until it finally settles under you. You are lying on top of this small cloud. The cloud lifts you into the air and you see the beach becoming smaller and smaller. Your body is becoming lighter and lighter. You are feeling warm, secure and relaxed.

Now the cloud descends, and your body is feeling more relaxed. As the cloud touches the beach, you are feeling warm, heavy and relaxed. Focus on your breathing. Use your cue word for 2 breathing cycles: RELAX. At the end of the second cycle, open your eyes. You should feel energised and ready for action.

Alternatively, picture a warm house in the middle of winter. Keeping your eyes closed, think about the house – is it a country house or a town house? Is it modern or old? What sort of plants are in the house? Can you hear the cold wind outside? Can you feel the warmth inside the house? Perhaps you can smell the aroma of your favourite food drifting from the kitchen. Move through each room of the house, concentrating on what you can see, hear, smell and feel before going on to the next image. Once you have spent a short time exploring, you should know your house so well that you could describe it to someone else.

Note that when you use relaxation imagery techniques, it is not the same as visualising with your eyes open. When visualising with your eyes open, you get a sharp, focused picture that remains steady. In contrast, mental images tend to be more fluid – more like ideas of what something looks like rather than a reproduction of reality.

Relaxation on the go

If stress symptoms occur in the workplace, then following some of the strategies below may help you manage your daily work stressors. Once you have finished a session of work, take a 5-minute break where you can:

- sit down and have a healthy snack, such as a piece of fruit;
- remove yourself from your working environment by going outside and walking around the block;
- find a quite place and practise the breathing, muscle relaxation and imagery techniques;
- withdraw to somewhere quiet, close your eyes and allow your body to rest; or
- if you are working from home, put on a favourite piece of music. Sit or lie down with your eyes closed and listen for a while.

Time management

Many of the daily hassles that cause us stress on a regular basis are caused by poor time management. Many people are simply not well organised, and trying to do too much in an unplanned fashion can generate the stress response. Characteristics of efficient time management include developing a long-term plan, prioritising and planning ahead, and using a yearly planner. Planning on a weekly basis involves filling in a weekly planner, using time slots wisely, being flexible, being realistic and seeking help. Common 'time thieves' are procrastinating, doing irrelevant tasks, failing to start a task, drifting off, being a perfectionist and putting tasks into the too-hard basket. Some easy-to-follow time-management tips include completing small tasks straight away, breaking tasks into sections and developing a goal-setting plan.

Goals are really useful for getting things done. They can be subjective, general objective, specific objective or outcome/performance-based. Guidelines for effective goal setting include:

- setting specific measurable goals;
- setting difficult but realistic goals;
- using short-range goals;
- developing performance-based rather than outcomes-based goals;
- setting positive rather than negative goals;
- identifying target dates;
- recording goals; and
- evaluating your goals.

Common problems that lead to failing to meet goals include setting too many goals, making goals too general, setting unrealistic goals and setting outcome goals. A goal-setting system allows you to assess your needs, set yourself long- and short-term goals, and evaluate your progress and adjust your goals weekly.

How to use the breathing, muscle relaxation, imagery relaxation and time-management techniques

You should try all these basic stress-management techniques to see which ones work best for you. Whatever you decide, an effective way of learning and performing the relaxation techniques is to make a tape or a script. Simply read out loud and record the scripts in each of the exercises above on a cassette player or using the record function on your phone, then practise the skills by playing and listening to the tape.

Ideally, you should try relaxing daily or at least 3 times per week. As you develop these relaxation skills, the protocols may be shortened and transferred to more realistic settings, which is called differential relaxation, though this may take weeks. Progression of differential relaxation could be: relaxing in a chair; relaxing in a car or train; relaxing during stressful situations during the day. Learning to monitor and control anxiety and tension can be achieved though a sound goal-setting system and well-structured stress-management skill sessions.

Exercise and stress reduction

The autonomic, cardiac and vascular changes occurring after participation in regular aerobic exercise are well documented. For example, low resting heart rate – bradycardia – typically occurs with regular aerobic exercise such as running. Resting heart rates of trained runners are often less than 50 beats per minute. Heart rate during an exercise session is also decreased after training.

These changes have prompted researchers to speculate that because regular aerobic exercise makes the body more efficient at handling exercise stress, then at the same time it will also produce a more efficient response to psychological stress. There is mixed evidence, however, to suggest that chronic physical activity may decrease the physiological response to stress in healthy individuals. The major finding appears to be that aerobic fitness is associated with slightly better heart-rate recovery to stress.[2]

A decrease in the stress response has been found in those few studies that have examined people at cardiovascular risk, such as people whose parents had hypertension or who have hypertension themselves, and we know that the blunted skeletal muscle bloodflow and increased blood pressure response to stress commonly found in the overweight and viscerally obese can be normalised with regular exercise.

These results have been derived mainly from studies using steady-state aerobic exercise, such as cycling, jogging and swimming, but the effects of other types of exercise, such as interval sprinting, on the stress response are poorly explored. We have shown that one session of interval sprinting, compared to one of steady-state exercise, produced a significantly greater impact on the autonomic nervous system assessed by heart rate and plasma catecholamine levels.[3] Regular interval sprinting training also resulted in a significant change in resting cardiovascular and autonomic function.[4]

Given that interval sprinting induces a significant acute cardiovascular response, it is possible that interval sprinting training may also produce greater adaptations to the stress response. Recently, we examined the effect of interval sprinting on the stress response; we found that 12 weeks of sprinting produced significant differences in cardiovascular and autonomic response during stress challenge.[5] Specifically, men who performed 12 weeks of interval sprinting experienced a significant reduction in heart rate during a psychological stress challenge. Exercisers compared to controls also showed decreased stiffness of their large arteries and increased muscle bloodflow during stress.

There are a number of other ways to use exercise to help relieve the stress in our lives. As mentioned earlier, regular involvement in exercise such as interval sprinting causes the body to adapt to both exercise and psychological stress. We know that exercisers have significantly less incidence of cardiovascular disease and stroke, but how much of this effect is due to a reduced stress response is unknown. Another way of using exercise to buffer the stress response is to use it as a 'time-out': after a busy morning at work, having a 50-minute jog around a pleasant park at lunchtime may distract an individual from the stress of work. Similarly, participating in 20 minutes of interval sprinting while listening to invigorating music may also direct people's thoughts away from daily stressors. However, more research on the stress-reducing capacity of interval sprinting is needed.

What is sleep?

Most human behaviours have an obvious purpose. For example, we eat to provide energy for the body and drink water to supply fluid in and around the cells. Up to 30% of a person's life may be spent in sleep, however the physiological function of sleep is unknown. The 2 main hypotheses to explain why we have to sleep are restoration and protection. The restoration hypothesis suggests that we sleep to restore the energy depletion that occurs during the previous day. However, approximately the same amount of energy is expended while sitting and sleeping. Moreover, bedridden people sleep more than normal people. The protective hypothesis suggests that our nervous system carries hard-wired behavioural patterns; because we lack adequate night sensors, it is safer to sleep at night. Whatever the reason for sleeping, it is known that lack of sleep or poor-quality, non-refreshing sleep has a bad effect on health; after the common cold, sleep problems are the second-biggest health complaint, and there are over 50 identified sleep disorders.

People experiencing regular sleep disruption typically possess greater body and belly fat than people who sleep well. Sleep-deprived people also have greater problems losing fat after a diet or exercise intervention. Differences in the number of hours of sleep also influence body composition, as it has been shown that people who sleep less tend to be overweight.[6] Disrupted sleep may change the balance between satiety hormones that control hunger, as sleeping 5 hours per night results in greater ghrelin and less leptin levels compared to sleeping 8 hours. Leptin is a hormone that is secreted by fat cells and tells the brain that we have had enough to eat. In contrast, ghrelin is secreted from the lining of the gut and makes us hungry. Thus, sleep deprivation affects body fat accumulation because it makes us hungrier. Increased resting cortisol levels have also been found in people who experience lack of sleep. Thus, sleeping well is very important for helping the body spend longer in fat-burning rather than fat-storing mode.

The effect of sleep on health

Together with healthy eating, exercise and stress-management, sleep is now acknowledged as one of the 4 pillars of a healthy lifestyle. Poor-quality sleep can have a major effect on people's emotional state and their ability to concentrate and remember. Also, sleep disorders such as obstructive sleep apnoea contribute to hypertension development, type 2 diabetes and cardiovascular disease. Poor-quality sleep also causes decreases in productivity and an increase in workplace and driving accidents. An Australian report estimated that sleep disorders incurred a cost of over $5 billion per year.

There are many sleep disorders but the major ones are insomnia, narcolepsy, sudden infant death syndrome (SIDS) and sleep apnoea. Insomnia is characterised by difficulty falling asleep, waking up frequently, waking up too early and non-refreshing sleep. Sleep apnoea is when a person's breathing pauses during sleep. Individuals who have this condition are often unaware of their problem, have daytime sleepiness and fatigue, regularly snore and their throat muscle and tongue relax too much when sleeping.

Obese people tend to develop sleep apnoea more than normal-weight people, and it is more common

Measuring the quality of your sleep

The quality of your sleep can be assessed by using the test below. Answer the 6 questions, using a score between 1 and 4 for each question, and then add up your total. If you score less than 4 points, then you have poor-quality sleep and need to take action to improve your sleep.

1 = Not at all **2 = Sometimes**
3 = Fairly regularly **4 = All the time**

1. I have difficulty falling asleep within 15 minutes

2. I wake up in the middle of the night or early morning

3. I constantly feel too hot or too cold in bed

4. I wake up too early and can't get back to sleep

5. I regularly have bad dreams

6. On waking, I feel tired and do not feel refreshed

TOTAL

Interpreting your score:
6-9 points: good-quality sleep
10-12 points: moderately good-quality sleep
13-18 points: moderately poor-quality sleep
19-24 points: very poor-quality sleep

in men and in older individuals. Sleep apnoea patients typically have low blood-oxygen levels and increased stress hormone levels, higher blood pressure, greater incidence of heart attack, stroke and heart failure, more irregular heartbeats and increased work-related or driving accidents. The treatment for sleep apnoea involves positive airway pressure, mouthpieces, sleeping on one's side, oxygen, practising wind instruments, surgery and lifestyle change.

The effect of sleep on belly fat

A study published in the journal of *Sleep* found that sleep duration was related to increases in belly fat.[7] Results showed that people sleeping less than 5 hours a night gained more belly fat over 5 years, compared to people sleeping over 6 hours a night. Short sleepers experienced a 32% gain in belly fat, compared to a 13% gain for people who slept 6 or 7 hours each night. Individuals who slept at least 8 hours of sleep each night showed a 22% increase in belly fat for both men and women over the 5-year period.

Another study, carried out by the National Sleep Foundation in 2003, found that older men and women who slept poorly experienced greater type 2 diabetes development. There was a higher incidence of sleep problems in older adults who were obese or overweight, though about half of older adults exercised 3 or more times per week. The more that older people exercised, the less likely they were to report poor-quality sleep.

Sleep onset

Change in body temperature directly affects sleep onset. Body core temperature refers to the temperature in organs deep inside the body, such as the brain and spinal cord, whereas skin temperature is the temperature of the extremities of the body, such as the hands and feet. When body core temperature increases, people tend to be more active and awake. In contrast, when body core temperature goes down, they become sleepy.

A hormone called melatonin is produced by the pineal gland at night and initiates the sleep cycle by lowering body core temperature. Melatonin levels are reduced by ageing, by exposure to bright light and by lack of sleep. Consequently, older adults, those exposed to bright light and shift workers or those who do not get an adequate amount of sleep are likely to have reduced melatonin and a reduced ability to sleep well.

Studies have shown that, after taking paracetamol or aspirin right before sleep, people fall asleep more quickly. This affect is attributed to these drugs' ability to lower the body's core temperature. A research group at the University of Pittsburgh also showed that when the front of insomniacs' heads were cooled by a special cooling cap, the insomniacs slept as well as normal sleepers. As discussed below, hot, sweaty exercise may enhance the onset and quality of sleep by lowering core temperature.

Strategies for increasing the quality of sleep are:

- keeping regular hours;
- cutting out stimulants;
- ensuring you have a good-quality bed;
- not smoking late (or at all);
- not drinking late;
- setting a 'worry time' before sleeping; and
- exercising regularly in the late afternoon.

Tips for sleep preparation include:

- Avoid vigorous exercise directly before bedtime. Leave at least 2 hours between aerobic exercise and going to bed.
- Gently stretching for 1 to 2 minutes before bed may help you relax.
- Eat your evening meal at least 1 hour before bed, but don't go to bed hungry, as being hungry may keep you awake.
- Listen to the radio (not TV) as you lie in bed

with your eyes closed. This is an effective way of falling asleep.

- Have a warm (not hot) bath last thing at night.

- Drink warm herbal tea half an hour before bedtime. Chamomile is particularly relaxing.

- Avoid alcohol, caffeine and nicotine for at least 5 hours before bed.

- Establish a steady bedtime routine with a regular time to go to bed and to rise.

- Try not to discuss work or domestic problems in bed. Treat your bed as your sanctuary where work issues are not allowed.

Exercise and sleep

Exercise has an important role to play in enhancing the quality of sleep. Hot, sweaty aerobic exercise in the late afternoon has been shown to result in better quality sleep. Sauna baths (thermal therapy) have also been shown to improve sleep quality if performed in the late afternoon. The exercise mechanism may be the same as that in thermal therapy. During hot, sweaty exercise, body core temperature increases, but after exercise has stopped, body core temperature starts to decrease. As mentioned previously, when body core temperature goes down, people become sleepy. Thus, exercise may increase sleep quality by influencing sleep centres in the brain such as the hypothalamus and sleep hormones such as melatonin. Exercise in the morning, however, does not appear to affect sleep onset or quality. There are a number of things to consider when using exercise to increase the quality of your sleep:

- Exercise in the late afternoon.
- Use vigorous aerobic exercise that induces sweating.
- Participating in resistance exercise does not appear to improve sleep quality.
- The effect of interval sprinting on sleep quality is unknown.

*

It's clear that high levels of stress and not enough sleep can severely affect our health, and that we can improve our health by improving stress-management and poor-quality sleep. The key points to keep in mind are:

- People who have high levels of daily stress and who sleep poorly tend to have higher levels of cortisol in their blood and typically have more belly fat.

- **There are a number of dietary and behavioural strategies you can use to reduce the effects of stress and to enhance sleep quality.**

- **Relaxation techniques and interval sprint training can help you cope with stress, while moderately vigorous aerobic exercise in the late afternoon is more effective than less vigorous exercise for sleep enhancement.**

Chapter 6
A 6-week belly fat loss program

As has been previously discussed, many of the key health benefits of interval sprinting occur after 6 weeks. Just 1 hour of interval sprinting each week for 6 weeks can significantly decrease belly fat, as measured by waist circumference, and insulin resistance. Interval sprinting has also been shown to significantly increase leg and abdominal muscle mass and aerobic fitness. We think interval sprinting is one of the 4 pillars of health; the other pillars include healthy eating, controlling the effect of daily stress and ensuring good-quality sleep. It is clear that making changes in these other areas will further enhance the health benefits of interval sprinting. This chapter contains a 6-week lifestyle program for someone who requires change in each of those 4 areas. The goals for each component are listed, together with examples of a weekly program.

To begin the program, first complete the self-tests that assess your fitness levels (Appendices A and B, pages 200–202) and add them to those you completed earlier for your body composition (Appendix E, page 208), your diet (Chapter 4, page 115), your amount of daily stress (Chapter 5, page 162) and your sleep quality (Chapter 5, page 182). It's a good idea to photocopy these pages so you can continue to assess your performance as the program progresses. Keeping records will help you to adjust the program, according to your individual assessment, your personal preferences and time availability.

Developing an interval sprinting program

Choose a form of exercise, such as cycling or sprint skipping, from those described in Chapter 3. If you choose the stationary bike, select a pedalling rate and resistance to help determine your exercise intensity. Other forms of interval sprinting, such as swimming, may only involve determining rate. Determine how many times per week you want to sprint, at what intensity and for how long each session.

It is important to perform interval sprinting with the correct technique and at the optimal intensity. Details on developing the best interval sprinting program for your level of fitness and health are described in Chapter 3 (page 75).

Interval sprinting goals

- Have your health checked before undertaking interval sprinting.
- Determine the mode, rate and exercise intensity preferable for you.
- Gradually increase the length and intensity of your training during the first 2 weeks.

Examples of light, moderate and hard interval sprinting programs that can be performed in the morning, at lunch-time, and in the evening are described in Chapter 3 (pages 75–112).

Adding an interval sprinting exercise program for the upper body

A lower- and upper-body interval sprinting protocol on alternate days is likely to result in a better total body workout. For example, a session of rowing, boxing or rope skipping as a combination or individually for 20 minutes is likely to result in extra health benefits. Of course, if you can only do 60 minutes of exercise a week, then the 3 20-minute sessions on the stationary bike is optimal. This would still only add up to 1 hour of interval sprinting per week, plus 24 minutes of warm-up and cool-down. An example of a lower- and upper-body interval sprinting program at a light intensity is described on page 192.

	Before sprinting	**Time of day: 6-8am**	**Pedal rate & resistance**	**Information to record**
Mon	Drink water or green tea	20 minutes LifeSprints on the bike	90rpm at 0.5kg, with 50rpm recovery	Weight and fat, exercise heart rate and RPE
Tues	Drink water or green tea	20 minutes rowing, skipping or boxing	See pages 89-90	Exercise heart rate and RPE
Wed	Drink water or green tea	20 minutes LifeSprints on the bike	90rpm at 0.5kg, with 50rpm recovery	Exercise heart rate and RPE
Thurs	Drink water or green tea	20 minutes rowing, skipping or boxing	See pages 89-90	Exercise heart rate and RPE
Fri	Drink water or green tea	20 minutes LifeSprints on the bike	90rpm at 0.5kg, with 50rpm recovery	Exercise heart rate and RPE
Sat	Rest day			
Sun	Drink water or green tea	20 minutes rowing, skipping or boxing	See pages 89-90	Exercise heart rate and RPE

Example of a lower- and upper-body interval sprinting program at a light intensity (rpm = revolutions per minute; RPE = rating of perceived exertion).

Adopting the Mediterranean eating plan

To gain the best results from your interval training program, you should make an assessment of your current diet by completing the diet assessment in Chapter 4 (page 115) or by using a free online dietary analysis program like www.nutridiary.com.

If you have an unhealthy diet, then follow the Mediterranean plan for 6 weeks as outlined in Chapter 4. Most people will not need to count calories on this diet. After 3 weeks you should feel more energy and less tiredness. The recipes for Monday's and Tuesday's meals are included in Chapter 4 (page 113); please consult the endnotes for recipes for the week's remaining meals.

Controlling daily stress

As well as an interval sprinting and heathy eating program, it's important to limit the amount of stress in your life for optimum belly fat loss. As discussed in Chapter 5, individuals exposed to stressors may increase their belly fat stores due to elevated cortisol and insulin levels.

Regular exercise, breathing, muscle relaxation, imagery and time-management skills are likely to be helpful in reducing the negative effects of daily stressors. Poor-quality sleep also results in elevated cortisol levels and increased belly fat, thus stress-management

	Breakfast	**Lunch**	**Dinner**
Mon	Scrambled egg on toast, green or black tea, or water, 1 piece of whole fruit	Curried vegetables (recipe, p.140), green or black tea, or water, mixed fruit	Roasted salmon and asparagus, wine*, dark chocolate, fruit, nuts
Tues	Fruit salad with yoghurt, green or black tea, or water	Spicy burrito (recipe p.140), green or black tea, or water, mixed fruit	Lemon caper chicken with couscous, wine, fruit
Wed	Cereal with fruit, green or black tea, or water	Fish tacos with avocado and salsa,[1] green or black tea, or water, mixed fruit	Shrimp and vegetable quinoa fried rice,[6] wine, fruit nuts
Thurs	Scrambled egg on toast, green or black tea, or water, 1 piece of whole fruit	Tuna Tahini salad,[2] green or black tea, or water, mixed fruit	Tandoori chicken with fresh vegetables and rice,[7] wine, fruit
Fri	Fruit salad with yoghurt, green or black tea, or water	Garden vegetable wrap,[3] green or black tea, or water, mixed fruit	Grilled halibut with avocado sauce,[8] wine, fruit, nuts
Sat	Cereal with fruit, green or black tea, or water	Black bean salad,[4] green or black tea, or water, mixed fruit	Steak stir fry with vegetables,[9] red wine, dark chocolate, fruit
Sun	Fruit salad with yoghurt, green or black tea, or water	Satay chicken with steamed vegetables[5] green or black tea, or water, mixed fruit	Cod poached in tomato sauce with spinach,[10] wine, fruit, nuts

An example of 1 week of a Mediterranean eating plan

*Limit is 1 glass for women and 2 for men

techniques and sleep quality enhancement strategies need to be implemented.

Below is an example of a practice schedule for stress-management enhancing strategies, for implementation alongside interval sprinting and healthy eating.

Mon	20 minutes of muscle relaxation and breathing
Tues	10 minutes of imagery
Wed	20 minutes of muscle relaxation and breathing
Thurs	10 minutes of imagery
Fri	20 minutes of muscle relaxation and breathing
Sat	
Sun	

Stress-management practice schedule

Enhancing quality of sleep

If after completing your sleep quality assessment in Chapter 5 (page 165) you find that your sleep needs to be improved, then you can work your way through the suggested techniques and tips to see which ones work best for you. For example, you could set a goal of creating a pre-sleep routine, perhaps aiming to drink a cup of herbal tea and do 10 minutes of relaxation using the imagery technique every night.

Consuming the appropriate nutrients before and after interval sprinting

As discussed in Chapter 4 (page 156), digesting nutrients before, during and after interval sprinting affects fat burning. Consuming sugary drinks and eating protein snacks before exercise will impede fat burning and reduce long-term fat loss, while other nutrients can enhance fat burning after and during exercise. Ingesting green tea before exercise significantly increases fat burning during the hour after a session of interval sprinting.

Exercising in the morning, before eating, is the ideal time to burn more fat during exercise and to put the body into fat-burning mode. Drink water or good-quality green tea before, during and after exercise, but try to refrain from eating for at least 45 minutes after exercise. If you can only exercise in your lunch hour, the best strategy would be to not eat anything for 3 hours before exercising.

*

The 4 pillars of a healthy lifestyle have now been described, and suggested programs for interval sprinting, healthy eating, stress-management and sleep quality have been outlined. An example of a weekly program involving these 4 critical behaviours is: 20 minutes of bike interval sprinting, 3 times per week (pages 98–101);

Mediterranean eating every day (page 125); daily stress-management technique practice (pages 162–179); and the use of sleep quality enhancement strategies every night (pages 179–188).

Try it for 6 weeks, recording your results at the same time each week, and discover the difference just 1 hour of interval training a week can make.

Monitoring progress

As described in Chapter 3 (pages 75–112), to monitor your progress, you need to record a certain amount of information. This information could include the following:

- heart-rate response during exercise (pages 75–79, 108)

- heart-rate response during the 4-minute cool-down (page 93)

- pedal rate during bike exercise (page 93)

- pedal resistance during bike exercise (page 93)

- rating of perceived exertion during exercise (page 91)

- weight and/or body fat change (page 22)

- waist circumference change (page 26)

- abdominal width change (page 27)
- waist skinfold site change (page 28)
- mid-thigh circumference change (page 31)
- lower leg circumference change (page 31)
- diet assessment (page 115)
- daily stress level assessment (page 165)
- quality of sleep assessment (page 182)

What to expect

We and other research groups have shown that because interval sprinting imposes greater loads on all 3 muscle fibre types (slow, intermediate and fast-twitch), its impact on total and belly fat, aerobic fitness, insulin resistance and muscle mass is both greater and quicker than that of other forms of exercise.[11] As the average person does not have the equipment or expertise to directly measure these health changes, indirect and simple measures can be utilised. We have shown that many of these positive changes can occur after 6 weeks – just 18 sessions – of properly performed interval sprinting on a stationary bike.

Over the last 10 years, we have witnessed a consistent increase in the amount of studies examining different aspects of interval sprinting in research labs in

Australia, the USA, Europe and Asia. The results have been impressive and consistent. We have no doubt that, for reducing belly fat and decreasing insulin resistance, interval sprinting is the premier form of exercise. Given that it produces these effects with at least half the exercise time, it is ideal for those of us who live busy lives.

We have given you a substantial amount of information in this book, but it's up to you how you use it: for some, the information on how to do interval sprinting may be enough; for others, changing their whole lifestyle may be appealing.

We believe that embarking on an interval sprinting program will significantly enhance your quality of life, and may even prevent or decrease the effect of a number of lifestyle diseases. And it only takes 6 weeks.

Appendix A
The Cooper 12-minute walk/run test

This 12-minute fitness test is a convenient way to assess aerobic fitness. The test assumes there is a reasonable relationship between the distance a person can run or walk in 12 minutes and their maximum aerobic fitness. The aerobic values achieved through this easy field test can be compared with those of people of the same age and gender. Test results, however, are affected by motivational factors; thus, being less or more motivated to run or walk could influence test results.

To perform the Cooper 12-minute walk/run test, you have to run or walk as far as you can in 12 minutes. It is usually completed on a running track, and a stopwatch is required to make sure you walk/run for 12 minutes exactly. This test can be demanding, so make sure you have a physician's clearance.

First, warm-up for 8–10 minutes, then run or walk as

far as you can in 12 minutes. After you have completed the test, compare your results to the norms below.

Age	Excellent	Above Average	Average	Below Average	Poor
Males 20-29	>2.8km	2.4-2.8km	2.2-2.4km	1.6-2.2km	<1.6km
Males 30-39	>2.7km	2.3-2.7km	1.9-2.3km	1.5-1.9km	<1.5km
Males 40-49	>2.5km	2.1-2.5km	1.7-2.1km	1.4-1.7km	<1.4km
Males 50+	>2.4km	2.0-2.4km	1.6-2.0km	1.3-1.6km	<1.3km
Females 20-29	>2.7km	2.2-2.7km	1.8-2.2km	1.5-1.8km	<1.5km
Females 30-39	>2.5km	2.0-2.5km	1.7-2.0km	1.4-1.7km	<1.4km
Females 40-49	>2.3km	1.9-2.3km	1.5-1.9km	1.2-1.5km	<1.2km
Females 50+	>2.2km	1.7-2.2km	1.4-1.7km	1.1-1.4km	<1.1km

Norms for the 12-minute walk/run aerobic fitness test.

Source: Cooper.[1]

Appendix B
Submaximal aerobic fitness test

Complete this test before beginning your 6- week interval sprinting program. Set up your stationary bike as per the instructions in Chapter 3 (page 88). The aim is to complete 3 bouts of continuous cycling for a total of 10 minutes: 4 minutes, 3 minutes and another 3-minute stage. Record your heart rate and rating of perceived exertion (RPE) (see page 91) at the end of the 3 exercise stages. Typical heart rates should be around 100 beats per minute during stage 1, 115 beats per minute during stage 2 and 130 beats per minute during stage 3 for people aged in their 20s and 30s. Typical heart rates should be around 90 beats per minute during stage 1, 105 beats per minute during stage 2 and 120 beats per minute during stage 3 for people aged in their 40s and 50s. Your heart rate should not go above 140 beats per minute during the test.

Collect your data and then plot your heart rate data on the graph in Appendix C (page 205).

Male

Name: Date:

	Pedal rate	Pedal resistance	Heart rate	RPE	Collection time
Stage 1 4 minutes	60rpm	1.0kg			At end of stage
Stage 2 3 minutes	60rpm	1.5kg			At end of stage
Stage 3 3 minutes	60rpm	2.0kg			At end of stage
Cool down 4 minutes	40rpm	0.5kg			

Female

Name: Date:

	Pedal rate	Pedal resistance	Heart rate	RPE	Collection time
Stage 1 4 minutes	60rpm	0.5kg			At end of stage
Stage 2 3 minutes	60rpm	1.0kg			At end of stage
Stage 3 3 minutes	60rpm	1.5kg			At end of stage
Cool down 4 minutes	40rpm	0.5kg			

Appendix C
Monitoring heart-rate change using the submaximal fitness test

If the submaximal test is repeated using the same workloads and under the same climatic conditions, the 3 heart rates at the 3 different pedal resistances will be lower if you have improved your aerobic fitness. Plotting your heart rates on this graph for a submaximal test repeated every 3 or 4 weeks should show a decrease in the heart-rate response. The decreased heart rate comes about because of increases in stroke volume and enhanced mitochondrial enzymes in the exercising muscles.

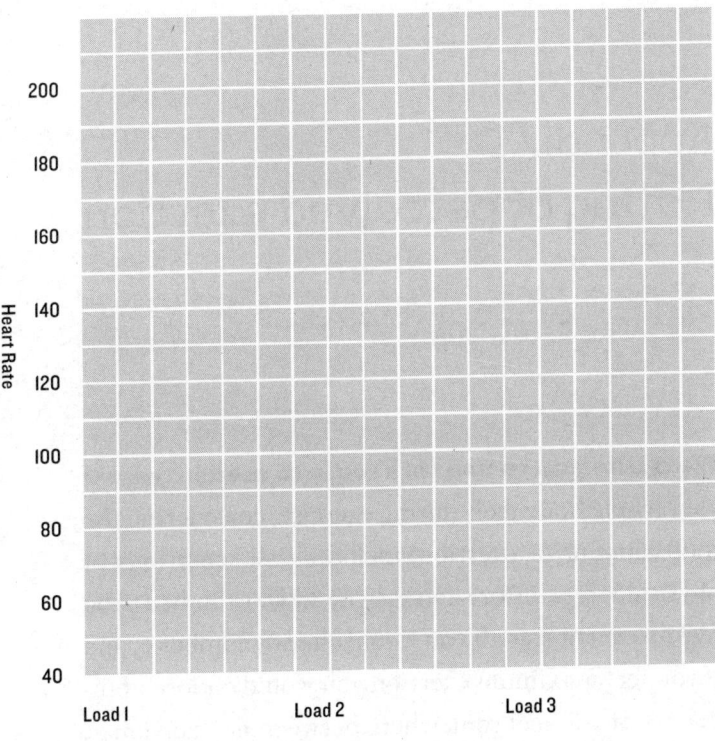

Appendix D
Rating of perceived exertion

We'd like you to use this scale to measure how your whole body feels during exercise, considering the total amount of exertion, including all sensations of physical stress, effort and fatigue in your body. If you feel no exertion at all you would choose number 6, and if you feel maximum exertion you would choose number 20. If you feel somewhere between no exertion at all and maximum exertion, then you would choose a number between 6 and 20. Remember, this scale refers to your whole body exertion, not your legs specifically. You can use any number from the scale to describe how you feel, which is likely to change during your exercise time.

Borg's RPE Scale

6	No exertion at all
7	Extremely light
8	
9	Very light
10	
11	Light
12	
13	Somewhat hard
14	
15	Hard (Heavy)
16	
17	Very hard
18	
19	Extremely hard
20	Maximal exertion

Appendix E
Body composition recording form

This form contains variables that you can record weekly or twice weekly on a non-exercise day, allowing you to chart your progress to see what body composition variables change. Having someone else take the measure reduces error and it is best if 2 measures are recorded and the average value documented. Instructions for collecting these measures can be found in Chapter 1 (pages 5–33).

20 x 3

	Value 1	Value 2	Average
Name:			Date:
Session number:		Time of day:	Temperature:
Weight (kg)			
Waist circumference (cm)			
Abdominal width (cm)			
Waist skinfold (mm)			
Upper leg circumference (cm)			
Lower leg circumference (cm)			

Comments:

Appendix F
Interval sprinting recording form

This form contains variables that you can record before, during and after each interval sprinting session. By recording these data you can chart your progress to see if you improve. You can also use this information to adjust your pedal rate and pedal resistance as you increase your fitness and become accustomed to interval sprinting.

20×3

	Pedal rate sprint	Pedal rate recovery	Pedal resistance	Heart rate	RPE	Collection time
Warm-up: 4 min						At end of warm-up
5 min						During 5th minute
10 min						During 10th minute
15 min						During 15th minute
20 min						During 20th minute
Cool-down: 4 min						During 24th minute

Name:

Date:

Session number:

Time of day:

Temperature:

Pre-exercise drink: Water   Green tea

Comments:

Appendix G
Weekly progress form

This form contains variables that you can record separately from the interval sprinting session, including body composition and cardiovascular data. Record your cholesterol, triglyceride (trig), low-density cholesterol (LDL) and high-density lipoprotein (HDL) levels, if you have them. By recording these data you can track any changes.

20 x 3

Name:		Date:		Time of day:	
Body composition		**Cardiovascular**		**Fitness, stress, sleep, fatigue, diet**	
Variable		**Variable**		**Variable**	
Weight		Resting heart rate		Submax test heart rate	
Body fat %		Systolic BP		Stress levels	
Muscle mass		Diastolic BP		Sleep quality	
Waist circumference		Cholesterol		Med eating score (see page 127)	
Waist skinfold		Trigs			
Abdominal width		LDL			
Mid-thigh circumference		HDL			
Lower leg circumference					

Comments:

Acknowledgements

I would like to thank the many subjects in our studies who carried out these interval sprinting programs. Thanks also go to the many medical students who made a significant contribution to data collection. A team of PhD students organised and ran these studies, including Mehrdad Heydari, Ehsan Ghareman and Sarah Dunn. The team at Black Inc. provided invaluable help that made this book possible. Finally, I would like to thank my wife, Yati, who made a significant contribution to the book, both from her published studies and with her editorial help and suggestions.

Resources

In this section there are listed a number of useful books and websites that provide information for helping with a lifestyle change based on interval sprinting exercise and healthy eating.

Exercise

LifeSprints

LifeSprints is an interval sprinting music program based on the 8-second/12-second principle: sprinting for 8 seconds followed by easy pedalling for 12 seconds. LifeSprints music is available on iTunes. A website has been developed by the author and includes lots of information regarding belly fat and up-to-date references on interval sprinting: www.bellyfatresearch.com.

Exercise physiologists

In Australia, exercise physiologists are trained to design lifestyle-change programs for unhealthy and diseased individuals. More information on exercise physiologists and their governing organisation, Exercise & Sports Science Australia (ESSA), can be found at www.essa.com.au.

An excellent introductory text for exercise physiology is: W. D. McArdle, F. I. Katch & V. L. Katch, *Exercise Physiology: Energy, nutrition, and human performance* (seventh edition), Lipponcot, Williams & Wilkins, Baltimore, 2010.

Nutrition and diet

C. Wheeler & D. A. Welland, *The Complete Idiot's Guide to Belly Fat Weight Loss*, Alpha Books, New York, 2012. This book contains useful information on diet and Mediterranean recipes.

J. Brand-Miller, K. Foster-Powell, J. McMillan & R. J. Robertson, *Low GI diet: 12-week weight-loss plan*, Hachette, Sydney, 2012. This book contains useful information on glycemic index and diet.

K. Tessmer & S. Green, *The Complete Idiot's Guide to the Mediterranean Diet*, Alpha Books, Indianapolis, 2010. This book contains lots of Mediterranean recipes.

The National Weight Control Registry (www.nwcr.ws). The NWCR is a group of people who are monitored to help show what is most important for long-term weight control.

Mark Hyman, *Ultrametabolism: The simple plan for automatic weight loss*, Schwartz Publishing, Melbourne, 2006. This book provides an excellent overview of health and metabolism.

Australian Dietary Guidelines (www.nhmrc.gov.au/guidelines/publications/n55). This site provides evidence-based guidelines for lifestyle change involving nutrition and physical activity.

Websites containing recipes and information on coconut:
www.freecoconutrecipes.com
www.coconutresearchcenter.org

Website containing information on protein in plants:
www.gentleworld.org/10-protein-packed-plants

Websites containing a range of Mediterranean recipes:
www.lifestylefood.com
www.eatingwell.com
www.allrecipes.com

Stress-management

Brian Luke Seaward, *Managing Stress: Principals and strategies for health and well-being*, Jones & Bartlett, Burlington, 2004.

A. Elkin, *Stress-management for Dummies*, Alpha Books, New York, 2013.

Joan Borysenko, *Minding the Body, Mending the Mind*, Addison-Wesley Publishing, Reading, 1987.

Stress Management: how to reduce, prevent, and cope with stress: www.helpguide.org/mental/stress_management_relief_coping.htm. www.mindtools.com is another website that contains a range of resources for dealing with stress.

M. Davies, E. Eshelman & M. McKay, *The Relaxation and Stress Reduction Workbook*, New Harbinger, Oakland, 2008. This self-help workbook contains lots of practical tips for reducing stress.

Sleep quality

Woodson Merrell, *The Source*, Free Press, New York, 2000. A good overview of fatigue and energy and how it is related to sleep.

Colin Espie, 'How to improve your sleep', *The Guardian*, 2011; see www.guardian.co.uk/lifeandstyle/2011/jan/29/how-to-improve-your-sleep.

WellnessMama.com, 'How to improve your sleep naturally'; see www.wellnessmama.com/4936/how-to-improve-sleep-naturally.

Endnotes

Chapter 1: Understanding Belly Fat

1. Australian Bureau of Statistics (2010), Measures of Australia's Progress, 2010 (cat. no. 1370.0), www.abs.gov.au /ausstats/abs@.nsf/mf/1370.0
2. Misra, A, & Khurana, L (2008), 'Obesity and the metabolic syndrome in developing countries', Journal of Clinical Endocrinology & Metabolism, 93, S9–S30.
3. Ford, ES, Li, C. Zhao, G, & Tsai, J (2011), 'Trends in obesity and abdominal obesity among adults in the United States from 1999-2008', International Journal of Obesity, 35, 736–743.
4. Jacobs, EJ, Newton, CC, Wang, Y, Patel, AV, McCullough, ML, Campbell, PT, Thun, MJ, & Gapstur, SM (2010), 'Waist circumference and all-cause mortality in a large US cohort', Archives of Internal Medicine, 170(15), 1293–1301.
5. Children's Sizing Report Launch, Shape GB: Measuring the nation, www.shapegb.org/childrens_sizing_report_launch.
6. Heitmann, BL (2009), 'Thigh circumference and risk of heart disease and premature death: prospective cohort study', British Medical Journal, 339:b3292, www.bmj.com/content/339/bmj.b3292.
7. Spalding, KL, Arnerm, E, Westermarkm PO, Bernard, S, Buchholz, BA, Bergmann, O, Blomqvist, L, Hoffstedt, J, Näslund, E, Britton, T, Concha, H, Hassan, M, Rydén, M, Frisén, J, & Arner, P (2008), 'Dynamics of fat cell turnover in humans', Nature, 453, 783–787.
8. Wajchenberg, BL (2000), 'Subcutaneous and visceral adipose tissue: their relation to the metabolic syndrome'. Endocrine Reviews, 21(6), 697–738.

9. O'Keefe, JH, Bybee, KA, & Lavie, CJ (2007), 'Alcohol and cardiovascular health: the razor-sharp, double-edged sword', Journal of the American College of Cardiology, 50, 1009–1014.
10. Katzmarzyk, PT, Bray, GA, Greenway, FL, Johnson, WD, Newton, RL, Ravussin, E, Ryan, DH, Smith, SR, & Bouchard, C (2010), 'Racial differences in abdominal depot-specific adiposity in white and African American adults', American Journal of Clinical Nutrition, 91(1), 7–15.
11. Després, JP, Couillard, C, Gagnon, J, Bergeron, J, Leon, AS, Rao, DC, Skinner, JS, Wilmore, JH, & Bouchard, C (2000), 'Race, visceral adipose tissue, plasma lipids, and lipoprotein lipase activity in men and women', Arteriosclerosis, Thrombosis, and Vascular Biology, 20, 1932–1938.
12. Fujimoto, WY, Newell-Morris, LL, Grote, M, Bergstrom, RW, & Shuman, WP (1991), 'Visceral fat obesity and mortality: NIDDM and atherogenic risk in Japanese American men and women', International Journal of Obesity, 15, Supp 2, 41–44.
13. Banerji, MA, Faridi, N, Atluri, R, Chaiken, RL, & Lebovitz, HE (1999), 'Body composition, visceral fat, leptin, and insulin resistance in Asian Indian men', Journal of Clinical Endocrinology & Metabolism, 84(1), 137–144.
14. Anand, SS, Tarnopolsky, MA, Rashid, S, Schulze, KM, Desai, D, Mente, A, Rao, S, Yusuf, S, Gerstein, HC, & Sharma, AM (2011), 'Adipocyte hypertrophy, fatty liver and metabolic risk factors in South Asians: the Molecular Study of health and risk in ethnic groups (molSHARE)'. PLoS ONE, volume 6, Issue 7, e22112, www.plosone.org/article/info%3Adoi%2F10.1371%2Fjournal.pone.0022112.
15. Canoy, D, Wareham, N, Luben, R, Welch, A, Bingham, S, Day, N, & Khaw, KT (2005), 'Cigarette smoking and fat distribution in 21,828 British men and women: a population-based study', Obesity Research, 13, 1466–1475.
16. Hou, X, Lu, J, Weng, J, Ji, L, Shan, Z, Liu, J, Tian, H, Ji, Q, Zhu, D, Ge, J, Lin, L, Chen, L, Guo, X, Zhao, Z, Li, Q, Zhou, Z, Shan, G, Yang, Z, Yang, W, & Jia, W (2013), 'Impact of waist circumference and body mass index on risk of cardiometabolic disorder and cardiovascular disease in Chinese Adults: A National Diabetes and Metabolic Disorders survey', PLoS ONE, 8(3): e57319. doi:10.1371/journal.pone.0057319.
17. Raffaitin, C, Féart, C, Le Goff, M, Amieva, H, Helmer, C, Akbaraly, TN, Tzourio, C, Gin, H, & Barberger-Gateau, P (2011), 'Metabolic syndrome and cognitive decline in French elders: the Three-City

Study', Neurology, 76(6), 518–525.
18. Guallar-Castillón, P, Sagardui-Villamor, J, Banegas, JR, Graciani, A, Fomés, NS, López Garcia, E, & Rodríguez-Artalejo, F (2005), 'Waist circumference as a predictor of disability among older adults', Obesity, 15(1), 233–244.
19. Larsson, SC, & Wolk, A (2007), 'Obesity and colon and rectal cancer risk: a meta-analysis of prospective studies', American Journal of Clinical Nutrition, 86, 556–565.
20. World Health Organization (2004), 'Appropriate body-mass index for Asian populations and its implications for policy and intervention strategies', Lancet, 363(9403), 157–163.
21. Alberti, KG, Zimmet, P, & Shaw, L (2005), 'The Metabolic Syndrome — a new worldwide definition', Lancet, Sep 24–30, 366, 1059–1062.

Chapter 2: The effect of exercise on belly fat and health

1. Wu, T, Gao, X, Chen, M, & van Dam, RM (2009), 'Long-term effectiveness of diet-plus-exercise interventions vs. diet-only interventions for weight loss: a meta-analysis', Obesity Reviews, 10, 313–323.
2. Ohkawara, K, Tanaka, S, Miyachi, M, Ishikawa-Takata, K, & Tabata, I (2007), 'A dose- response relation between aerobic exercise and visceral fat reduction: systematic review of clinical trials', International Journal of Obesity, 31, 1786–1797.
3. Ismail, I, Keating, SE, Baker, MK, & Johnson, NA (2012), 'A systematic review and meta-analysis of the effect of aerobic vs. resistance exercise training on visceral fat', Obesity Reviews, 13, 68–91.
4. Mourier, A, Gautier, JF, De Kerviler, E, Bigard, AX, Villette, JM, Garnier, JP, Duvallet, A, Guezennec, CY, & Cathelineau, G (1997), 'Mobilization of visceral adipose tissue related to the improvement in insulin sensitivity in response to physical training in NIDDM. Effects of branched-chain amino acid supplements', Diabetes Care, 20(3), 385–391.
5. Trapp, G, Chisholm, D, Freund, J, & Boutcher, SH (2008), 'The effects of high-intensity intermittent exercise training on fat loss and insulin levels of young women', International Journal of Obesity, 32, 684–691.
6. Dunn, SL (2009), 'Effects of exercise and dietary intervention on

metabolic syndrome markers of inactive premenopausal women', Doctoral dissertation, University of New South Wales, 20109, http://unswroks.unsw.edu.au/vital/access/manager/Repository/unsworks:345.

7. Heydari, M, Freund, J, & Boutcher, SH (2012), 'The effect of high-intensity intermittent exercise on body composition of overweight young males', Journal of Obesity. Volume 2012, Article ID 480467, doi: 10.1155/2012/480467.

8. Boutcher, SH (2011), 'The effects of high intensity intermittent exercise on fat loss', Journal of Obesity, 2011; 2011: 868305. Epub 2010 Nov 24.; Ohkawara, et al., loc. cit.; Ismail, et al., loc. cit.

9. Peterson, MD, Sen, A, & Gordon, PM (2010), 'Influence of resistance exercise on lean body mass in aging adults: A meta-analysis', Medicine and Science in Sports & Exercise, 43, 249–258.

10. Trapp, et al., loc. cit.; Dunn, loc. cit.; Heydari, et al., loc. cit.

11. Thivel, D, Isacco, L, Rousset, S, Boirie, Y, Morio, B, & Duché, P (2010), 'Intensive exercise: A remedy for childhood obesity', Physiology & Behavior, doi:10.1016/j.physbeh.2010.10.011.

12. Tan, M., Chan, R.M.F., Boutcher, Y.N., & Boutcher, S.H. (in press), 'Effects of high-intensity intermittent exercise on plasma postprandial triacylglycerol in sedentary young women', International Journal of Sport Nutrition & Exercise Metabolism.

13. Boutcher, SH, & Dunn, SL (2009), 'Factors that may impede the weight loss response to exercise-based interventions', Obesity Reviews, 10, 671–680.

14. Heydari, et al., loc. cit.

15. Blair, SN (2009), 'Physical inactivity: the biggest public health problem of the 21st century', British Journal of Sports Medicine, 43, 2114–2120.

16. Trapp, et al., loc. cit.

17. Dunn, loc cit.; Heydari, et al., loc. cit.

18. Kuk, JL, Janiszewski, PM, & Ross, R (2007), 'Exercise, visceral adipose tissue, and metabolic risk', Current Cardiovascular Risk Reports, 1, 254–264.; Trapp, et al., loc. cit.; Dunn, loc. cit.

19. Meyer, K, Samak, L, Schwaibold, M, Westbrook, S, Hajric, R, Beneke, R, Lehmann, M & Roskamm, H (1997), 'Interval training in patients with severe chronic heart failure: analysis and recommendations for exercise procedures', Medicine & Science in Sports and Exercise, 29, 306–312.

20. Munk, PS, Staal, EM, Butt, NB, Isaksen, K, & Larsen, AI (2009), 'High-intensity interval training may reduce in-stent restenosis

following percutaneous coronary intervention with stent implantation A randomized controlled trial evaluating the relationship to endothelial function and inflammation', American Heart Journal, 158, 734–741.

21. Moholdt, TT, Amundsen, BH, Rustad, LA, Wahba, A, Løvø, KT, Gullikstad, LR, Bye, A, Skogvoll, E, Wisløff, U, & Slørdahl, SA (2009), 'Aerobic interval training versus continuous moderate exercise after coronary artery bypass surgery: A randomized study of cardiovascular effects and quality of life', American Heart Journal, 158, 1031–1037.

22. Nilsson, BB, Westheim, A, & Risberg, MA (2008), 'Long-term effects of a group-based high-intensity aerobic interval training program in patients with chronic heart failure', American Journal of Cardiology, 102, 1220–1224.

23. Wisløff, U, Støylen, A, Loennechen, JP, Bruvold, M, Rognmo, Ø, Haram, PM, Tjønna, AE, Helgerud, J, Slørdahl, SA, Lee, SJ, Videm, V, Bye, A, Smith, GL, Najjar, SM, Ellingsen, Ø, & Skjaerpe, T (2007), 'Superior cardiovascular effect of aerobic interval training versus moderate continuous training in heart failure patients: a randomized study', Circulation, 115(24), 3086–3094.

24. Rognmo, Ø, Hetland, E, Helgerud, J, Hoff, J, & Slørdahl, S (2004), 'High intensity aerobic interval exercise is superior to moderate intensity exercise for increasing aerobic capacity in patients with coronary artery disease', European Journal of Cardiovascular Prevention & Rehabilitation, 11, 216–222.

25. Ernst, C (2009), 'The role of exercise interval training in treating cardiovascular disease risk factors', Current Cardiovascular Risk Reports, 3, 296–301.

26. Vogiatzis, I, Terzis, G, Nanas, S, Stratakos, G, Simoes, DCM, Geogiadou, O, Zakynthinos, S, & Roussos, C (2005), ' Skeletal muscle adaptations to interval training with patients with advanced COPD', CHEST, 128, 3838–45.

27. ibid.

28. Kortianu, EA, Nasis, IG, Spetsioti, ST, Daskalakis, AM, & Vogiatzis, I (2010), 'Effectiveness of interval exercise training in patients with COPD', Cardiopulmonary Physical Therapy Journal, 21, 12–19.

29. Tjønna, AE, Lee, SJ, Rognmo, Ø, Stølen, TO, Bye, A, Haram, PM, Loennechen, JP, Al-Share, QY, Skogvoll, E, Slørdahl, SA, Kemi, OJ, Najjar, SM, & Wisløff, U (2008), 'Aerobic interval training versus continuous moderate exercise as a treatment for the metabolic syndrome: a pilot study', Circulation, 118(4), 346–354.

30. Praet, SFE, Jonkers, RA, Schep, G, Stehouwer, CDA, Kuipers, H, & van Loon, LJ (2008), 'Long-standing insulin-treated type 2 diabetes patients with complication respond well to short-term resistance and interval exercise training', European Journal of Endocrinology, 158, 163–172.
31. Little, JP, Gillen, JB, Percival, ME, Safdar, A, Tarnoplosky, MA, Punthakee, Z, Jung, ME, & Gibala, MJ (2011), 'Low-volume high-intensity interval training reduces hyperglycemia and increases muscle mitochondrial capacity in patients with type 2 diabetes', Journal of Applied Physiology, 111, 1554–1560.
32. Bussau, VA, Jones, TW, Ferreira, LD, & Fornier, PA (2006), 'A novel approach to counter an exercise-mediated fall in glycemia in individuals with type 1 diabetes', Diabetes Care, 29, 601–606.
33. Guelfi, KJ, Ratnam, N, Smythe, GA, Jones, TW, & Fornier, PA (2007), 'Effect of intermittent high-intensity compared with moderate exercise on glucose production and utilization in individuals wth type 1 diabetes', American Journal of Physiology, Endocrinology & Metabolism, 292(3), E865–870.
34. Kessler, HS, Sisson, SB, & Short, KR (2012), 'The potential for high-intensity interval training to reduce cardiometabolic disease risk', Sports Medicine, 42(6), 489–509.
35. Slørdahl, SA, Wang, E, Hoff, J, Kemi, OJ, Amundsen, BH & Helgerud, J (2005), 'Effective training for patients with intermittent claudication', Scandanavian Cardiovascular Journal, 39, 244–249.
36. Adams, J (2006), 'High-intensity interval training for intermittent claudication in a vascular rehabilitation program', Journal of Vascular Nursing, 24, 46–49.
37. Trapp, et al., loc. cit.; Heydari, et al., loc. cit.
38. Coker, RH, Williams, RH, Kortebein, PM, Sullivan, DH, & Evans, WJ (2009), 'Influence of exercise intensity on abdominal fat and adiponectin in elderly adults', Metabolic Syndrome & Related Disorders, 7, 363–368.
39. O'Leary, VB, Marchetti, CM, Krushman, RK, Stetzer, BP, Gonzalez, F, & Kirwan, JP (2006), 'Exercise-induced reversal of insulin resiatnce in obese elderly is associated with reduced visceral fat', Journal of Applied Physiology, 100, 154–158.
40. Tjønna, AE, Stølen, TO, Bye, A, Volden, M, Slørdahl, SA, Odegård, R, Skogvoll, E, & Wisløff, U (2009), 'Aerobic interval training reduces cardiovascular risk factors more than a multi treatment approach in overweight adolescents', Clinical Science, 116, 317–326.
41. Boutcher, 'The effects of high intensity intermittent exercise on fat

loss', loc. cit.
42. Mourier, et al., loc. cit.
43. Tjonna, et al., loc. cit.

Chapter 3: The Interval sprinting belly fat loss program

1. Bracken, RM, Linnane, DM, & Brooks, S (2009), 'Plasma catecholamine responses to brief intermittent maximal intensity exercise', Amino Acids, 36, 209–217.
2. Trapp, EG, Chisholm, DJ, & Boutcher, SH (2007), 'Metabolic response of trained and untrained women during high-intensity intermittent cycle exercise', American Journal of Physiology, 293(6), R2370–R2375.
3. Robertson, R.J (2004), Perceived exertion for Practitioners: rating effort with the OMNI picture system, Champaign, IL: Human Kinetics.
4. Heydari, M, & Boutcher, SH (2013), 'Rating of perceived exertion after 12 weeks of high-intensity intermittent sprinting', Perceptual Motor Skills, 116, 1, 340–351.
5. Trapp, et al., 'Metabolic response of trained and untrained women during high-intensity intermittent cycle exercise', loc. cit.
6. ibid.
7. Bracken, et al., loc. cit.
8. Nevill, ME, Holmyard, DJ, Hall, GM, Allsop, P, van Oosterhout, A, Burton JM, & Nevill, AM (1996), 'Growth hormone responses to treadmill sprinting in sprint- and endurance-trained athletes', European Journal of Applied Physiology, 72, 460–467.

Chapter 4: Dieting, nutrients and belly fat

1. O'Keefe, JH, & Cordain, L (2004), 'Cardiovascular disease resulting from a diet and lifestyle at odds with our Paleolithic genome: how to become a 21st-Century hunter-gatherer', Mayo Clinical Proceedings, 79, 101–108.
2. www.freecoconutrecipes.com; www.coconutresearchcenter.org
3. Engler, MM, & Engler, MB (2006), 'Omega-3 fatty acids: role in cardiovascular health and disease', Journal of Cardiovascular Nursing, 21(1), 7–24.
4. Campbell, TC, & Campbell, TM (2006), The China Study: The Most

Comprehensive Study of Nutrition Ever Conducted And the Startling Implications for Diet, Weight Loss, and Long-term Health, BenBella Books, Dallas, TX.
5. www.gentleworld.org/10-protein-packed-plants/
6. Fife, B (1999), Saturated Fat May Save Your Life. Piccadilly Books, Ltd., Colorado Springs, CO.
7. Micha, R, Wallace, SK, & Mozaffarian, D (2010), 'Red and processed meat consumption and risk of incident coronary heart disease, stroke, and diabetes mellitus', Circulation, 121, 2271–2283.
8. www.gentleworld.org/10-protein-packed-plants/
9. Mann, T, Tomiyama, AJ, Westling, E, Lew, AM, Samuels, B, & Chapman, J (2007), 'Medicare's search for effective obesity treatments: Diets are not the answer', American Psychologist, April 62, 220–233.
10. Chaston, TB, & Dixon, JB (2008), 'Factors associated with percent change in visceral versus subcutaneous abdominal fat during weight loss: findings from a systematic review', International Journal of Obesity, 32, 619–628.
11. de Lorgeril, M, & Salen, P (2006), 'The Mediterranean-style diet for the prevention of cardiovascular diseases', Public Health Nutrition, 9(1A), 118–123.
12. de Lorgeril, M (1998), 'Mediterranean diet in the prevention of coronary heart disease', Nutrition, 14(1), 55–57.
13. Trichopoulou, A, Costacou, T, Bamia, C, & Trichopoulos, D (2003), 'Adherence to a Mediterranean diet and survival in a Greek population', New England Journal of Medicine, 348, 2599–2608.
14. Mann, et al., loc. cit.
15. Tsai, AG & Wadden, TA (2005), 'Systematic review: An evaluation of major commercial weight loss programs in the United States', Annals of Internal Medicine, 142, 56-66.
16. Klem, ML, Wing, RR, McGuire, MT, Seagle, HM, & Hill JO (1997), 'A descriptive study of individuals successful at long-term maintenance of substantial weight loss', American Journal Clinical Nutrition, 66, 239–246.
17. Hsu, TF, Kusumoto, A, Abe, K, Hosado, K, Wang, M-F, & Yamamoto, S (2006), 'Polyphenol-enriched oolong tea increases fecal lipid excretion', European Journal of Clinical Nutrition, 60(11), 1330–1336.
18. Bravo, E, Napolitano, M, & Botham, K (2010), 'Postprandial lipid metabolism: The missing link between life-style habits and the increasing incidence of metabolic diseases in western countries?' The Open Translational Medicine Journal, 2, 1–13.

19. Tan, et al., loc. cit.
20. O'Keefe, JH, Gheewala, NM, & O'Keefe, JO (2008), 'Dietary strategies for improving post-prandial glucose, lipids, inflammation, and cardiovascular disease, alcohol, and cardiovascular health', Journal of the American College of Cardiology, 51, 249–255.
21. Ghahramanloo, E (2012), 'Effects of green tea extract and high intensity intermittent exercise on fat metabolism', Doctoral dissertation, University of New South Wales. http://unswroks.unsw.edu.au/vital/access/manager/Repository/unsworks: 345
22. Venables, MC, Hulston, CJ, Cox, HR, & Jeukendrup, AE (2008), 'Green tea extract ingestion, fat oxidation, and glucose tolerance in healthy humans', American Journal of Clinical Nutrition, 87(3), 778–784.
23. Van Proeyen, K, Szlufcik, K, Nielens, H, Pelgrim, K, Deldicque, L, Hesselink, M, Van Veldhoven, V, & Hespel, P (2010), 'Training in the fasted state improves glucose tolerance during fat-rich diet', Journal of Physiology, 111, 4289–4302.
24. Martins, C, Morgan, LM, Bloom, SR, & Robertson, MD (2007), 'Effects of exercise on gut peptides, energy intake, and appetite', Journal of Endocrinology, 193, 251–258.
25. Sim, AY, Wallman, KE, Fairchild, TJ, & Guelfi, KJ (2013), 'High-intensity intermittent exercise attenuates ad-libitum energy intake', International Journal of Obesity, Jun 4. Doi: 10.1038/ijo. Epub ahead of print.
26. White, LJ, Dressendorfer, RH, Holland, E, McCoy, SC, & Ferguson, MA (2005), 'Increased caloric intake soon after exercise in cold water', International Journal of Sport Nutrition and Exercise Metabolism, 15(1), 38–47.

Chapter 5: Reducing daily stress and enhancing sleep quality

1. Borysenko, J (1987), 'Minding the body, mending the mind', Reading, MA: Addison-Wesley Publishing.
2. Forcier, K, Stroud, LR, Papandonatos, GD, Hitsman, B, Reiches, M, Krishnamoorthy, J, & Niaura, R (2006), 'Links between physical fitness and cardiovascular reactivity and recovery to psychological stressors: A meta-analysis', Health Psychology, 25, 723–739.
3. Bracken, et al., loc. cit.

4. Heydari, M, Boutcher, YN, & Boutcher, SH (2013,) 'The effects of 12-week high-intensity intermittent exercise training on cardiovascular and autonomic measures during mental and physical stress', International Journal of Psychophysiology, 87(2), 141–146.
5. Heydari, M, Boutcher, YN, & Boutcher, SH (2013), 'The effects of 12-week of high intensity intermittent exercise training on resting cardiovascular and autonomic function', Journal of Clinical Autonomic Control, 23(1), 57–65.
6. Patel, SR, & Hu, FB (2008), 'Short sleep duration and weight gain: a systematic review', Obesity, 16, 643–653.
7. Hairston, KG, Bryer-Ash, M, Norris, JM, et al. (2010), 'Sleep duration and five-year abdominal fat accumulation in a minority cohort: The IRUS Family study', Sleep, 33, 289–295.

Chapter 6: A 6-week belly fat loss program

1. Fish tacos with avocado salsa recipe: www.taste.com.au/recipes/16763/fish+tacos+with+avocado+salsa.
2. Tuna tahini salad recipe: www.mamavation.com/2012/03/tahini-tuna-salad.html.
3. Garden vegetable wrap recipe: spryliving.com/recipes/garden-vegetable-wrap.
4. Black bean salad recipe: www.simplyrecipes.com/recipes/black-bean-salad.
5. Satay chicken with steamed vegetables recipe: www.taste.com.au/recipes/10415/satay+chicken+with+steamed+vegetables.
6. Shrimp and vegetable quinoa fried rice recipe: www.queenofquinoa.me/2012/09/shrimp-vegetable-quinoa-fried-rice.
7. Tandoori chicken with fresh vegetables and rice recipe: www.sbs.com.au/food/recipe/121/Tandoori-chicken.
8. Grilled halibut with avocado sauce recipe: www.avocadocentral.com/avocado-recipes/Grilled-Halibut-with-Avocado-Chipotle-Cream-Sauce.
9. Steak stir fry with vegetables recipe: www.tasteofhome.com/recipes/Vegetable-Steak-Stir-Fry.
10. Cod poached in tomato sauce with spinach recipe: www.thescrumptiouspumpkin.com/2012/11/02/cod-poached-in-tomato-sauce-with-spinach-capers-and-pine-nuts.
11. Trapp, et al., 'The effects of high-intensity intermittent exercise training on fat loss and insulin levels of young women', loc cit.; Dunn,

loc. cit.; Boutcher, 'The effects of high intensity intermittent exercise on fat loss', loc. cit.

Appendix A

1. Cooper, KH (1968), 'A means of assessing maximal oxygen uptake', Journal of the American Medical Association, 203, 201–204.

Index

abdominal fat, 27
abdominal muscle, 8
abdominal width, 27
aerobic exercise
   assessment, 202
   effect on belly fat, 34
alcohol, 16, 130
animal proteins, 120
appetite, 44

beans, 129
belly fat
   what is it? 8
   health risks, 20
   measurement, 22
belly fat factors
   age, 15
   alcohol, 16, 130
   ethnicity, 17
   exercise, 36, 39
   sleep, 183
   smoking, 19
   stress, 164
bike, 88
bioelectrical impedance, 25
body fat, 8
body mass index, 23
breakfast
   recipes, 137

breathing techniques, 167

C-reactive protein, 12
cocoa, 130
caffeine, 149
capsaicin, 149
cardiovascular disease, 8, 9
carbohydrates
   simple, 116
   complex, 116
chocolate, 130
Cooper 12-min walk/run test, 200
cortisol, 10, 162

dark chocolate, 130
depression, 63
diets, 123
digestion
   carbohydrate, 116
   fructose, 116
dinner
   recipes, 142
drinks
   alcohol, 16, 130
   caffeine, 149
   green tea, 148
   water, 196

eating questionnaire, 115

epinephrine, 11, 84, 148
ethnicity, 17
exercise and appetite, 158
exercise physiologists, 217

fat, 117
fat in the blood, 154
fat mobilisation, 11
fat-storing hormones, 10
fat-burning hormones, 11
fat loss and aerobic exercise, 41
fibre, 122
fish oils, 119
free weights, 36
fresh vegetables, 135
frozen vegetables, 136
fructose, 116
fruit, 131

genes, 12
ghrelin, 180
glucose, 10
green tea, 148
goal setting, 175
growth hormone, 85

heart-rate measurement
  palpitation, 78
  monitor, 79
heart rate during sprinting, 76, 91
high-fructose corn syrup, 116
hunter-gatherer lifestyle, 114

imagery techniques, 171
inflammation, 8, 126
insoluble fibre, 122
insulin resistance, 54
intermittent claudication, 65
interval sprinting exercise
  what it is, 37
  how to do it, 86
  deciding on pedal rate, 89
  deciding on pedal resistance, 89
  optimal exercise heart rates, 91
  rating of perceived exertion, 91
interval sprinting and nutrition before, during and after, 156
interval sprinting mechanisms
  increased fat burning, 42
  increased muscle mass, 44
  decreased appetite, 44
  decreased postprandial lipemia, 46
interval sprinting modalities
  sprint cycling, 98
  sprint rowing, 101
  sprint walking, 101
  sprint stair climbing, 102
  sprint running, 103
  sprint arm ergometry, 103
  sprint boxing, 104
  sprint skipping, 104
  sprint swimming, 105
  sprint circuits, 105
interval sprinting music, 97
interval sprinting programs
  morning, 110
  lunchtime, 110
  evening, 111
interval sprinting response
  heart rate, 75
  hormones, 84
  catecholamines, 84
  growth hormone, 85
  rating of perceived exertion, 91
interval sprinting, special populations
  heart disease, 57
  chronic pulmonary disease, 59
  diabetes, 67
  depression, 63
  intermittent claudication, 65
  obesity, 67
  postmenopausal women, 69
  post-pregnant women, 70
  special population considerations, 72

job stress, 174
jogging, 35

lactate, 81
leg circumference measure, 31
leptin, 180
leafy vegetables, 135
lemon caper chicken, 143
LifeSprints, 97
lipoprotein lipase, 47
liver, 48, 116
lunch recipes, 140

maximal oxygen uptake test, 50
meat
  beef, 133
  chicken, 133
  turkey, 133
Mediterranean eating score, 127
Mediterranean eating plan, 125
  health benefits, 125
  how to switch, 144
  how to keep the fat off, 146
Mediterranean foods
  beans, peas, pasta, 129
  beverages, 130
  chocolate, 130
  dairy, 130
  fats, 131
  fruits, 131
  nuts and seeds, 133
  poultry and red meat, 133
  seafood, 134
  seasoning and spreads, 134
  vegetables, 135
  whole grains, 136
Mediterranean eating recipes
  scrambled eggs, 137
  fruits, nuts, yoghurt, 138
  curried vegetables, 140
  spicy burritos, 140
  roasted salmon, 142
  lemon caper chicken, 143
measuring fat, 22
measuring fitness, 202

metabolic syndrome, 61
muscle mass
  effect of aerobic exercise, 53
  effect of ageing, 16
  effect of diet, 53
  effect of interval sprinting, 52
music, 97

norepinephrine, 11, 84, 148
nutrients
  that burn fat, 148
  that impede fat burning, 151
  that reduce fat absorption, 152
nuts and seeds, 133

obesity
  incidence, 5
  children, 6
  factors, 9
oblique muscles, 100
olive oil, 119
optimal exercise heart rates, 91
organic pollutants, 153

pedal rate, 89
pedal resistance, 89
perceived exertion, 91
post-prandial lipemia, 154
power output, 88, 90
progress measurement, 106
protein, 120
pulmonary disease, 59

questionnaires
  eating style, 115
  physical activity levels, 14
  stress levels, 165
  sleep quality, 182

rating of perceived exertion, 79
recipes
  scrambled eggs, 137
  fruit, 138
  cereal, 138
  curried vegetables, 140

burrito, 140
salmon, 142
chicken, 143
red meat, 120
refined carbohydrates, 116
relaxation response, 167
resistance exercise
    belly fat, 36
    insulin resistance, 56
    muscle mass, 44
risks from belly fat, 20

salmon, 142
salt, 116, 122
satiety, 159
saturated fats, 117
seeds, 133
sugar, 116
sugar in the blood, 154
skeletal muscle, 44, 52
sleep
    sleep and health, 181
    sleep and belly fat, 183
    sleep enhancement, 184
    sleep and exercise, 186
soft drinks, 117
spices, 134
stress, 162
stress management
    breathing, 167
    coping, 166
    imagery, 171
    muscle relaxation, 169
stress and exercise, 177
stressors, 163
subcutaneous fat, 6
subcutaneous abdominal fat, 27
submaximal fitness test, 202

time management, 174
thyroid, 12
toxins, 153
transverse abdominis, 100
triglycerides, 147
Type 1 diabetes, 61
Type 2 diabetes, 61

upper-body interval sprinting, 103
unsaturated fats, 119

vegetables, 135
visceral fat, 7

waist circumference, 26
waist skinfold measure, 28
water, 149
watts, 90

yoghurt, 138